UNDERSTANDING
HEADACHES AND MIGRAINES

UNDERSTANDING HEADACHES AND MIGRAINES

DR J N BLAU

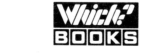

Published by Consumers' Association
and Hodder & Stoughton

Which? books are commissioned and researched by
The Association for Consumer Research
and published by Consumers' Association
2 Marylebone Road, London NW1 4DX and
Hodder & Stoughton, 47 Bedford Square, London WC1B 3DP

Edited by Dr Anthony Delamothe

Appendix compiled by Consumers' Association

Typographic design by Paul Saunders
Cover design by Ivor Claydon
Cover illustrations by courtesy of the Wellcome Institute
Library, London and Sally and Richard Greenhill
Illustrations by Stephen Player and Tony Richards

First edition April 1991
Copyright © 1991 Consumers' Association Ltd
Published by arrangement with The K S Giniger Company, Inc.,
250 W.57 St., New York, NY 10107, USA

This book is based on *The Headache and Migraine Handbook*
copyright © 1986 by J N Blau and originally published by Transworld
Publishers in association with The K S Giniger Company, Inc.

British Library Cataloguing in Publication Data
Blau, Joseph N. (Joseph Norman)
  Understanding headaches and migraines.
  1. Humans. Headaches
  I. Title II. Delamothe, A
  616.8491

ISBN 0 340 51862 6

Typeset by Litho Link Limited, Welshpool, Powys
Printed and bound in Great Britain by BPCC Hazell Books,
Aylesbury, Bucks. Member of BPCC Limited

CONTENTS

ABOUT THE AUTHOR

DR J N BLAU entered St Bartholomew's Hospital Medical College as a science scholar in 1947 and qualified in 1952. He was appointed consultant physician to the National Hospital for Nervous Diseases in London at 33 and later became neurologist to the Royal National Throat, Nose and Ear Hospital, London and Northwick Park Hospital, Harrow, Middlesex.

His migraine research began in depth in 1965. He was secretary of the Medical Advisory Panel of the Migraine Trust and later became Joint Honorary Director of the City of London Migraine Clinic.

He has researched prodromes, the earliest warning symptoms of migraine attacks, has studied how attacks are resolved and has investigated the 'hangovers' after attacks. He has also shown that fasting can precipitate migraines and diabetes can alleviate migraines; the study of blood vessels in the whites of the eyes during attacks has also formed part of Dr Blau's research.

He has recently studied headaches that occur after epileptic attacks, those due to insufficient sleep, and excess insulin in insulin-dependent diabetic patients.

He is honorary medical advisor of the British Migraine Association, has written papers in many learned medical journals, and is currently the chairman of the Medical Writers Group of the Society of Authors.

INTRODUCTION

ONLY ONE person in fifty can say, 'I have never had a headache in my life'. Yet behind the universal nature of this ailment lies a multiplicity of types and causes of headaches. This book aims to guide the reader through the various types of headache and their causes in order to assist in their self-diagnosis, treatment and avoidance.

Understanding Headaches and Migraines describes those rare types of headache for which professional medical attention should be sought: principally those of recent onset which are becoming more severe or happening at increasingly shorter intervals; or headaches that are accompanied by loss of consciousness or failing vision. Very few headaches are symptomatic of a serious disorder; for instance, most GPs, on average, encounter a case of a brain tumour only once in every seven-and-a-half to ten years. Nevertheless, headaches can often be debilitating, uncomfortable and distressing enough to cause the sufferer to seek advice and treatment.

The distinctive nature of migraines, both in the pattern and severity of their symptoms, together with the fact that over five million people in the UK alone suffer from them, obviously deserves major attention. Several chapters of the book are therefore devoted to this important subject. They detail the symptoms and pattern of migraine attacks, describe the factors that predispose some people to migraines and suggest methods of managing the condition, both with and without drugs.

Medical research on headaches and migraines is progressing at speed. The book takes a look at current research and some of the new theories being put forward in the study of this ailment. But, essentially, *Understanding Headaches and Migraines* is a practical guide to self-help – advisedly, as surveys suggest that two-thirds of headaches and migraines benefit from self-help.

As well as detailing conventional medical opinion on the treatment of headaches, the book includes an appendix on the variety of complementary therapies (compiled by Consumers' Association in association with the complementary therapy organisations), such as acupuncture, homoeopathy and the Alexander Technique, for those who wish to combat headaches without resorting to drugs.

PART 1

HEADACHES

CHAPTER 1

EVERYDAY HEADACHES

THIS CHAPTER includes headaches with simple causes. Unlike some dealt with later, these headaches are easily identifiable and, once understood, usually easily dealt with. Most of them relate to everyday activities, such as eating, and not eating, drinking, sleeping, shopping, and so on.

Hunger headaches

If we miss a meal, within a few hours we get a sinking feeling in the pit of our stomachs, which we recognise as hunger. If we continue without food, then that sinking feeling may be replaced by something more unpleasant, such as hunger pangs or a headache.

For a few people, a headache is the first sensation of hunger. This usually starts as a vague awareness in the forehead or on top of the head, which then progresses to actual discomfort or ache. Other tell-tale signs that all is not well, most obvious in children who aren't as good as adults in disguising their feelings, are high-spiritedness, irritability or, conversely, lethargy. In addition, many people feel cold when hungry and some go pale.

The remedy is simple: eat and within five to ten minutes the symptoms will disappear.

Although dealing with these headaches could hardly be simpler, recognising their cause may be difficult. Those who fast for religious purposes – for example, Orthodox Jews on the Day of Atonement (Yom Kippur) or Muslims during Ramadan – will have noticed that their headaches disappear as soon as they have eaten and will have no difficulty in making the connection. But not all hunger headaches follow such extremes as fasting. Delaying or missing meals or eating too little food may also be responsible for hunger headaches. Eating an apple or an orange when hungry might fill you up temporarily, but the calorie yield is low.

People differ widely in how much they need to eat. Some make do with one meal a day, others need three meals a day and additional snacks as well. (Some people even eat a meal at bedtime to prevent early morning headaches when blood sugar levels would otherwise be low.) It is important for you to work out your requirements, especially if your headaches seem to be cured by eating some food.

What can be done?

- Have a good breakfast to start the day. If you cannot face eating breakfast but are developing headaches during the morning, then try eating something like a sandwich with your morning tea or coffee.
- Don't substitute light snacks during the day for proper meals.
- If you are dieting, try to avoid losing weight quickly: rapid weight loss can lead to headaches.

CASE HISTORY

Trying to lose weight, a city banker cut down on lunch, taking only a light snack. Unfortunately, however, he began suffering from afternoon headaches. After he started eating more substantial lunches – lean meat, boiled potatoes and vegetables – he lost his headaches and found that he was no longer irritable when travelling home in the evening. Nor did he gain weight.

Headaches from nitrites and nitrates in food

Chemicals called nitrites and nitrates are added to meat, especially sausages, to make them look fresh and appetising. However, these chemicals also dilate blood vessels, which has led to their use in the treatment of angina. Patients using prescribed nitrates for angina occasionally complain of throbbing headaches that last for about five to ten minutes after taking their tablets, symptoms resulting from the dilation of the blood vessels supplying the brain. If they persist with this medication for angina, the headaches often disappear, or stop being troublesome, after a few weeks.

Chinese restaurant headaches

Headaches may occur after eating Chinese food which may be associated with other unpleasant symptoms, such as palpitations, dizziness, and tight feelings in the face, head and neck. Monosodium glutamate (MSG), a chemical used as a flavour enhancer in soya sauce (and other foodstuffs), has been blamed for this, although other factors may contribute.

For example, the food may arrive only after a long wait, and when it arrives it may be quite fatty (and fat slows down the absorption of food; consequently there is a further delay before glucose reaches the brain). Taken together, these two effects could add up to the conditions necessary for a hunger headache (p 15), regardless of how much monosodium glutamate is in the food.

What can be done?

- Eat a snack before you go out.
- Order a starter as soon as you arrive at the restaurant.
- Use the soya sauce sparingly, in case it contributes to your headache.
- MSG is used in other canned and bottled foods and sauces as well as a whole range of pre-packaged convenience foods. Those who suspect that MSG may be responsible for their headaches should think carefully about the content of their food as the MSG content may not be immediately obvious.

  US citizens get a much better deal than the British when it comes to food additives: some restaurants advertise themselves as 'MSG free' or are prepared to serve dishes that are MSG free.

Coffee withdrawal headaches

If coffee addicts (drinking 30 to 40 cups of coffee a day) try to stop their habit suddenly they may develop headaches. Drinking fewer cups but stronger coffee may produce the same problems.

What can be done?

- Do not let your coffee consumption increase to these levels, but if you do and you decide you want to reduce your intake, try stopping coffee completely or do it gradually.

Alcohol hangover headaches

'Morning after' headaches are universal, with most languages having their own special word or phrase to describe them. Perhaps the most expressive is the German *Katzenjammer*, which means wailing cats in your head.

You don't have to drink very much alcohol to get a hangover – some people find that drinking even a little on an empty stomach or when tired is sufficient.

Alcoholic drinks seem to vary in their potential to cause problems due to varying percentages of alcohol and the congeners (see below) added by the manufacturers to produce special flavours – for example, different varieties of whisky or brandy. One researcher found that vodka is least likely to produce a headache, while beer, sherry, port and brandy are most likely.

How does an alcoholic drink produce head and stomach disturbances eight to twelve hours later? No one knows, but as with all forms of headache, there is no shortage of suggestions.

Dehydration

Concentrated alcohol, as in fortified wine or liqueurs, sucks water from the blood and body tissues, which subsequently needs to be replaced. Many people find that they can prevent or reduce a hangover after a binge by drinking a pint of water before going to bed.

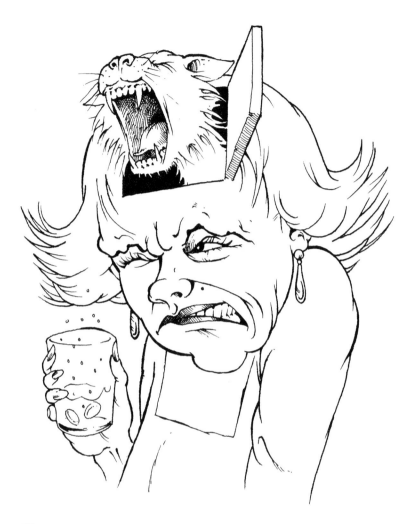

[Figure 1: *Katzenjammer* or 'wailing cats in your head'.]

Congeners

These additives give drinks their individual tastes (alcohol itself is tasteless). Some congeners are aromatic oils which, besides irritating the stomach, reach the brain where they may provoke headaches.

Low blood sugar

Low blood sugar may cause headaches. We know this from diabetics who develop headaches when their blood sugar is low from either taking too much insulin or eating too little food. Alcohol can affect the concentration of glucose in the blood (and therefore the brain) and thereby provoke a headache.

Low blood oxygen and high blood carbon dioxide

Mountaineers short of oxygen get headaches. Breathing oxygen may relieve headaches. Second World War pilots used to relieve their hangovers by breathing pure oxygen from masks normally used for flying at altitude. In the deep sleep of alcohol intoxication, when we breathe more shallowly, the blood oxygen level may fall and the carbon dioxide level rise – and a headache upon waking is the result.

What can be done?

- Discover those drinks that don't agree with you and avoid them.
- Find out how much you can drink and stay within your limits.
- Try drinking a pint of water (or milk) before going to bed – it may prevent your hangover.
- If you've found something that helps, such as aspirin or paracetamol and a cup of coffee, make sure you have them to hand.
- Don't be tempted to relieve your hangover with another drink: the 'hair of the dog' is a short cut to more serious drinking problems.

Headaches caused by a stuffy atmosphere, cigarette smoke or other smells

Smokers' own cigarette smoke, or that from someone else's cigarette, can result in headaches. The known health risks of smoking should encourage you to give up the habit. But if that is impossible, then find out how much you can tolerate, and which cigarettes, cigars or pipe tobacco suit you (but in moderation).

Petrol fumes, varnish, hairspray, insecticides and paint can all cause headaches. Smells do not have to be unpleasant: even walking through the perfume department of a large store or smelling the aroma of ground coffee may be enough to provoke headaches in a few people.

What can be done?

- Stay in well-ventilated places as much as possible. Keep a window open when driving or sleeping. Hotel bedrooms with fixed levels of central heating may present a problem – not just hot and stuffy, but dry as well. To combat the dryness try leaving some water in the wash basin to act as a humidifier.
- In offices a bowl of water or some flowers in a pot with moistened earth will act in the same way.
- At parties, where heat and alcohol may contribute to headaches, try to stand or sit near a window or door and arrive and leave a little early.

Headaches caused by the cold

Exposing the head to low temperatures can give rise to headaches. This can happen in two ways: either by eating or sucking something cold or by failing to protect the head in cold and windy weather.

Ice-cream headaches

Consuming any very cold food or drink quickly – with ice-cream the main culprit – can cause headaches. These are usually short-lived, lasting from 10 to 60 seconds, and are experienced as a pain or tightness in the forehead, at the top or back of the head, or all over. Occasionally, the pain is situated in the ears or behind the eyes. Experiments on volunteers whereby cold oxygen is delivered through the nose indicate that cold makes the muscles of the palate and nose tighten up into a painful spasm. Warming the oxygen stops the pain. Eating or drinking cold food slowly can help to avoid the problems of 'ice-cream headaches'.

CASE HISTORY

Novels and autobiographies often confirm medical views.

'He [the grandfather] loved to feed them large doses of ice-cream on summer afternoons, would laugh at them gently when they got the terrible sharp headache from eating too much too fast, and then give them a gentle lecture on gluttony.'

From: *The Ice-Cream Headache* by James Jones, Collins, 1968, London

Headaches from cold and windy weather

Just as ice-cream can cause the muscles of the palate and nose to tighten up, cold biting winds can cause the muscles of the head to contract painfully. Depending on which group of muscles is affected pain is felt in the forehead (*frontalis*), temples (*temporalis*), or back of the head (*occipitalis*). (See the diagram on page 34.)

What can be done?

- Treat your head as you would the rest of your body and wear appropriate headgear. Eskimos and Canadian trappers wear adequate protection on their heads; their solution may not be fashionable, but it works. Air is an excellent heat insulator – hence the value of a fur lining or a loose woollen-textured hat. Women, who generally have more hair, cope better than men, particularly middle-aged men with thinning hair.

Headaches from the weather and from dry winds

Some people get a headache when there are thundery conditions or a change in barometric pressure. In various parts of the world when dry winds blow (the Föhn of southern Europe is the best known) many people complain of headaches, associated with the sudden alteration in barometric pressure, which last until the winds have abated.

Name of wind	Region
chamsin or charav	Middle East
cinook	Canada
Föhn	Switzerland, southern Germany and Austria
Santa Anna	California
sirocco	Mediterranean
zonda	Argentina

What can be done?

- Nothing can be done about the weather, but simple analgesics such as aspirin or paracetamol may give some relief.

Exercise headaches

Some people start to exercise feeling perfectly well and then during (or more commonly after) exercise they develop a throbbing headache. These headaches usually affect both sides of the head and last from five minutes to 24 hours. One explanation of these may be that exercise dilates the blood vessels on the surface of the brain; another that the brain is short of glucose that has been diverted to the exercising muscles.

What can be done?

- Avoid exercising too strenuously, particularly in hot weather or at high altitudes.
- Try taking glucose tablets before and immediately after exercise, supplemented by some light food after changing.

Headaches associated with sexual activity

Several different kinds of headache are associated with sexual activity. The first is a dull ache at the back of the neck, which worsens as sexual excitement increases. Excessive contraction of the muscles of the head and neck are probably responsible for these headaches.

The second kind of headache occurs 'explosively' at orgasm and may be due to the sudden rise of blood pressure that occurs then.

Some people's headaches may be worse after orgasm, which may have the same explanation as exercise headaches (see p 23). If you experience headaches with an orgasm, you should seek medical advice.

Sleep headaches

Sleeping too long, too deeply, too little, or interrupted sleep may all give rise to headaches. Even if the mechanism is in doubt (even less is known about sleep than headaches), there are some obvious solutions.

Sleeping too long

About fifteen per cent of people develop a headache if they do not get up at their normal time. If this happens to you, it does not mean that you can never sleep in, but you will have to experiment. Allow an extra half an hour of sleep for a couple of weekends, then an extra hour for the next two, and so on, until you find out how much extra sleep you can tolerate before developing a headache.

Sleeping too deeply

This may explain why some people who don't have the opportunity to sleep 'well' during the week wake with a headache at the weekend. Remember that alcohol (see page 18) or sleeping tablets may each deepen sleep and leave you with a headache on waking.

Sleep deprivation

Headaches due to insufficient or interrupted sleep have previously been confused with 'tension headaches' (see page 31) and attributed to psychological upset. Recently, however, they have been recognised as something different. Unlike tension headaches, the headache of sleep deprivation responds well to simple analgesics, such as aspirin or paracetamol, or having a short nap.

CASE HISTORY

'Normally I need seven to eight hours' sleep. If I go to bed much later than usual on one or two successive nights, then I wake up with a dull ache in my forehead, which usually lasts about an hour. Sometimes it may last until lunchtime or even until I go to sleep at night.'

A 26-year-old nurse

Headaches from cinema, television and reading

Many people come out of the cinema with a headache, which may be due to their intense focusing on the screen. Having to focus continually for whatever reason – prolonged reading, staring at a computer or television screen, or peering down a microscope – may induce headaches. Driving long distances and having to concentrate on the road ahead may be a problem, too (see travel headaches, page 26).

What can be done?

- If headaches after a film are a problem, sit as far away from the cinema screen as possible. Similarly with television: don't sit too close, and keep a light on somewhere in the room. This should prevent excessive focusing on the screen, as you will tend to look at other parts of the room at intervals.
- If you think your eyes may be at fault, obtain professional advice. Your optician/ophthalmologist or general practitioner should be consulted.
- Some activities seem harmless enough in themselves and yet consistently trouble some people. How can something as

mundane as shopping or as exciting as travel bring on headaches? The answer is that they combine several features already discussed.

Shopping

If you shop when everyone else does, there will be a degree of bustle, tension and heat. All contribute to a stuffy, enclosed atmosphere, usually made less bearable by fluorescent lighting, particularly of the flickering variety. Research in Cambridge has shown that some fluorescent lights which flicker at a great frequency, and are therefore not perceived, can provoke headaches.

What can be done?

- Shop early before many other people are around. If a headache seems to develop while you are out shopping, stop and take one or two analgesic tablets, preferably with a cup of tea. (Never take tablets without a drink.) Then go home, eat lunch and take things quietly in the afternoon.

Travel

Journeys can induce headaches in diverse ways, each requiring different preventive action.

- Excitement or too much to do the night before may mean setting off with too little sleep.
- Hunger may be a factor: it may be too early to eat before leaving, or breakfast may be rushed, and the expected meal *en route* may be a long time coming.
- Travel sickness will keep you away from food; its effect will be the same as missing a meal (or two).
- Anxiety about making train, ferry or airport connections is perfect for triggering off a tension headache.
- If you are driving into the sun, the glare may give you a headache. Car drivers who keep a fairly fixed position are more at risk from neck tension than passengers.
- On aeroplane journeys there is the problem of pressurised cabins with insufficient oxygen. Often the air is very dry and

dehydration is also an important factor. Meals may be good, bad, or non-existent. Fear of flying and alcohol (often used to allay the fear) may both induce headaches.

What can be done?

- Work out which of the above factors apply to you. Careful planning and preparation help.
- If nausea is a problem take an anti-travel sickness tablet an hour before you set off. Your pharmacist will advise you on this (but beware of tablets that make you sleepy or impair concentration if you are going to drive a car).
- Don't forget the importance of food: consider taking some with you if you're not sure what will be available.
- A good pair of sunglasses and an anti-glare strip on the windscreen will help if you are sensitive to light. The driver is less likely to get carsick than the driven. This is not 'all in the head' – the driver is always focusing 20 or more yards ahead, whereas passengers are forever focusing at varying distances inside and out of the car. Furthermore, drivers 'move with the car' because they anticipate changes of speed over which they have control.

Headaches from tablets and other medication

A headache is quite a common side-effect of drugs. If you suddenly develop a headache after starting medication it is reasonable to assume that the two are related. Your instinct may be to stop the tablets, but before doing so you should discuss this with the doctor who prescribed them. The consequences of stopping a course of tablets may be much worse than the headaches themselves. In other cases a headache may be a symptom of the condition for which the tablets had been originally prescribed. If this is so, the headache has nothing to do with the tablets, and stopping these may make the headache worse. If you are being treated for high blood pressure or giant cell (temporal) arteritis (see page 52), be very wary of stopping your tablets or reducing their dose without taking medical advice.

WARNING

The oral contraceptive pill: some women cannot tolerate it because of the headaches it produces and they will need to find another method of contraception. Others on intermittent therapy may experience headaches only in their week off the pill, and they may be helped by the 'continuous pill' taken throughout the month.

Some of the drugs which have been found to provoke headaches in some people

amitriptyline
aspirin or paracetamol – 20 or more tablets a month
barbiturates
benzodiazepines (diazepam, nitrazepam, temazepam)
bromocriptine
dopamine
ephedrine
glyceryl trinitrate
imipramine
metoclopramide
monoamine oxidase inhibitors
oestrogen
    hormone replacement therapy (HRT) for women
    oral contraceptive pill
perphexiline
sulphonamides (including co-trimoxazole)
terbutaline
theophylline
tyramine

Drugs for high blood pressure (on starting or stopping treatment)
clonidine
hydralazine
labetalol
propranolol

Non-steroidal anti-inflammatory drugs
diclofenac
ibuprofen
indomethacin
ketoprofen
naproxen

Withdrawal of
amphetamine
benzodiazepines
caffeine
ergotamine
methysergide

Premenstrual headaches

Some women regularly have headaches two to seven days before their period is due. Two possible explanations have been given for this. The first is fluid retention, which some doctors think affects the brain as well as other tissues in the body premenstrually. Women who suffer from fluid retention complain that in the week before their period their breasts swell and become tender, their skirts feel tight, and rings may be difficult to remove from swollen fingers.

Weighing themselves they find that they have gained a few pounds. Diuretics, which help women pass more water and retain less fluid, can relieve these symptoms, although diuretics should always be used under medical supervision.

Other women who are prone to premenstrual headaches may not be troubled by fluid retention but feel irritable and touchy.

Allergy

Allergic explanations of disease, popular in the 1920s and 1930s, have made something of a comeback recently. Allergy (sometimes to some food constituent or additive) has been blamed for a whole range of symptoms, including headaches.

Many tests have been developed to check for allergy, but they lack precision. On skin testing, for example, some people seem to be allergic to a variety of different proteins, which when they inhale them (or eat them) cause no problems at all. The proof of allergy to particular foodstuffs is that you react badly on eating or drinking them. Other tests for allergy are *suggestive*, rather than *conclusive*.

What can be done?

If you suspect that something you are eating or drinking is causing your headaches, remove it from your diet for a specified period. It must be long enough for you to see whether its removal affects the frequency of your headache. If you have weekly headaches, stop the offending food for at least a month. Keep a diary of your headaches – if they do not disappear or become less frequent, then reintroduce that item and consider eliminating another. Only remove one food at a time: it will allow you to decide with greater certainty whether allergy is the problem.

CHAPTER 2

COMMON HEADACHES

HEADACHES may be related to certain activities (chapter 1) or some underlying anatomical problem (chapters 3 and 4). And then there are the rest – the vast majority. Experts differ over their actual order of importance but agree that tension headaches, muscle contraction headaches and migraines constitute 80 to 90 per cent of all headaches for which people seek further advice.

This chapter looks at these common headaches, together with a few others that are difficult to classify. Only brief sketches are given of migraine and cluster headaches. Migraines are sufficiently distinctive (and complicated) to warrant several chapters of their own (beginning with chapter 7, page 75), while further details of cluster headaches are given in chapter 13.

Tension headaches

People with tension headaches complain of a pressing or tightening sensation. They say it is like 'a weight on top of my head' or 'a band around my head as if I am wearing a tight hat'. They add that it is not so much a pain as an unpleasant awareness, pressure or discomfort. It may be difficult to date exactly when the headaches started.

Tension headaches can last minutes or several hours, but typically they are present all day. Some people wake with a headache, which persists until they fall asleep at night. The headaches affect both sides of the head and are usually constant, although stress and tiredness may make them worse. Ordinary physical exertion seems to have no effect. They don't interfere with eating and only rarely with work. Getting off to sleep and staying asleep may be difficult. (Headaches which are associated with vomiting or weight loss are not due to tension.)

Tension headaches take the pleasure out of life. Social life may be interfered with: these headaches stop some people going out and enjoying themselves.

What can be done – in the short term?

Sometimes relaxation, a hot bath, being busy at work or watching television may lessen the symptoms or even make them disappear. Analgesic tablets don't usually help as they are unable to affect or alter someone's mood.

What can be done – in the long term?

As their name suggests these headaches are thought to be due to tension. Being anxious or depressed may leave you feeling tense. Anxiety shows itself as an inability to relax or a difficulty in getting off to sleep. Depression makes you miserable – you lose interest in life and stop enjoying it. Sometimes you may even feel like crying for no reason at all.

Developing a headache in addition to anxiety or depression increases the original anxiety or depression because there may be the suspicion that the headaches are being caused by something sinister, such as a brain tumour. If the symptoms are as described for a tension headache your chances of having a brain tumour are almost nil.

Some treatment will still be needed for reducing tension (see chapter 5 and the appendix), but it is helpful if you try to work out what makes you tense. This is usually not very difficult, and once you have made the discovery you are in a better position to change things.

Muscle contraction headaches

The day after unaccustomed exertion, such as jogging, tennis, long-distance driving or gardening, the exercised muscles are stiff, which any movement makes worse. A hot bath helps and so does massaging the painful areas.

A similar process can affect the muscles of the head and neck if they are exercised in an unaccustomed way. The muscles can become tender, too, and the feelings may be just like a headache.

The head and neck have several well-developed muscle groups, concerned with expression, raising the eyebrows, frowning, opening and closing the jaw, and supporting and moving the head. Most head muscles are flat and are attached to the outside of the skull and the scalp (*galea aponeurotica*), a tendon situated at the top of the head immediately under the skin.

HEAD AND NECK MUSCLES

To feel the muscles of the head and neck contracting:
- put your hand on your forehead and move your eyebrows up and down (frontalis);
- put your fingertips on your temples and open and close your jaw (temporalis);
- put your fingers over the angle of your jaw and clench your teeth (masseters);
- put your hand high up on the back of your neck and move your head sideways and up and down (occipitalis and neck muscles).

Someone with a muscle contraction headache can usually localise the most painful spot with the tip of a finger. It will be over one of the muscles shown in figure 2, overleaf.

Muscle contraction headaches are more common in people who have to maintain a single position at work. Worst affected are secretaries typing for many hours a day, bench workers or computer operators who have to look down fixedly and long-distance drivers.

Wearing uncomfortable glasses may also give rise to pain in the forehead, because the muscles there are continually contracting to try to correct the discomfort.

These aches and pains are real, just as real as the pains you get in your shoulders and arms after carrying heavy shopping or suitcases. They originate in the muscles outside the skull and

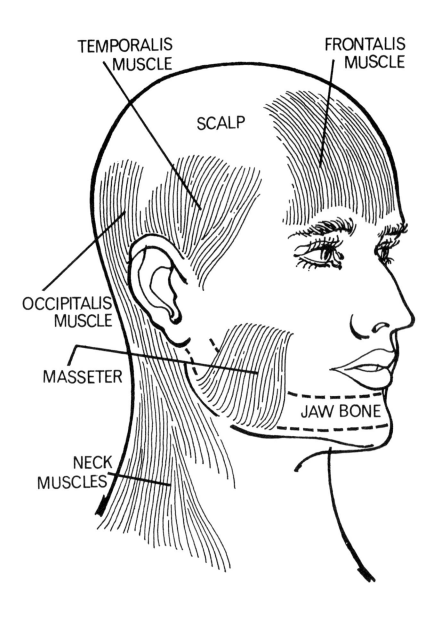

[Figure 2: Muscles of the face with which we move our eyebrows.]

therefore have nothing to do with the brain. Not knowing that, some people fear there is something wrong inside their heads so in addition to their muscle contraction headache they develop a tension headache from worrying about it.

Muscle contraction headaches are not the only cause of pains that seem to be coming from these muscles. Pains may be 'referred' there from other sites. In arthritis of the neck the upper neck muscles may be tender to touch and movements of the head and neck painful. With dental problems pain may be referred from the teeth to the jaw muscles. Referred pains are a common cause of headache, and the next chapter contains a fuller description of them.

Hyperventilation or muzziness headache

Hyperventilation headaches are most commonly due to anxiety. Individuals experience a range of symptoms that include a dizzy feeling and a mild headache. Some people overbreathe when anxious; others holding themselves tensely, breathe too shallowly for a while only to breathe more deeply when they relax. This results in a sensation inside the head, often interpreted as a headache.

It is simple to decide whether headaches are due to hyperventilation. If taking deep breaths for a minute or so brings on the usual headache, it is likely to be due to hyperventilation.

What can be done?

- Being aware of the harmless nature of these headaches often makes them easier to live with. Rebreathing into a paper bag covering your nose and mouth, so that you re-inhale the carbon dioxide just exhaled (for a short while), will reverse the symptoms as long as the bag is pressed tightly to the face.
- If symptoms remain a problem, a physiotherapist may be able to help you with the sort of breathing exercises taught to singers and public speakers. (They tend to hold their chests too tightly and experience the same symptoms as those described.) Some of the complementary therapies described in the appendix are useful in reducing stress.

Ice-pick headache

This type of headache can be identified as sudden sharp pains in various parts of the head, which feel as if a tiny sharp-ended hammer, like an ice-pick, is penetrating the scalp. Some sufferers describe the sensation as like a needle prick or as if the tissues under the skin were being nipped. These are very brief pains, lasting only seconds, and occur singly or as a series of stabs.

Because they appear to be more common in migraine sufferers the doctors who originally described them thought they were a variant of migraine, but they could also be due to muscle spasm (something like a stitch or a cramp in the legs, similar to the effect after running).

Fatigue or an over-awareness about the head could also be a cause of ice-pick headaches. Once again, sufferers may be reassured that nothing sinister is going on.

Migraine headaches – in brief

A migraine is a headache that lasts a good part of the day, or all day, *and* is accompanied by visual disturbances and/or stomach disturbances.

The typical features of migraines are:

- A migraine is not a headache that lasts a matter of minutes; nor does it persist for weeks or months. The normal duration is about a day. For some people an attack may be over in half a day; for others, attacks may last for one and a half, two, or even three days.
- Visual disturbances may take the form of an aura – a warning before the headache comes on – that lasts from 5 to 60 minutes. The aura may be a blind spot (*scotoma*), which enlarges or, more commonly, takes the form of flashing or flickering lights, which may be stationary or move across the field of vision. The more common visual disturbance is a sensitivity to light; in severe attacks migraine sufferers darken the room or wear dark glasses.
- Initially the stomach upset consists of a loss of appetite, which then gives rise to nausea and in some attacks to vomiting.

- During attacks the sufferers go pale and feel cold. If they lie down they cover themselves with blankets, even taking a hot-water bottle to bed or turn up the central heating.
- During an attack individuals become irritable and want to be left alone. Some have either a dislike or a heightened perception of smells.
- Most attacks end in sleep – usually a normal night's sleep – although some people manage to end their attacks by taking a nap for a few hours. Some find that vomiting ends their attack, which is the way attacks often end in children. Usually, however, attacks subside slowly, leaving a 'washed out' feeling the next day when a person still feels weak and has a limited tolerance for food as well as for physical and mental activity.

These and other features of migraines are discussed in much more detail in the second half of the book (see page 73).

Cluster headaches

As the name suggests, these headaches occur in clusters, that is, daily attacks for six to eight weeks followed by a period of freedom for a year or longer. Unlike other types of headache, cluster headaches affect men more frequently than women.

Typically, there is severe pain behind one, always the same, eye which wakens the sufferer in the early hours of the morning. After a few minutes the pain becomes very severe and the sufferer rises from his bed, paces the bedroom or sits down, cupping his head in his hands. The affected eye goes red, tears may stream from it and the nostril on the same side will either be blocked or discharge a clear fluid.

Attacks last from 20 minutes to two hours and may waken the sufferer with such regularity that the condition was once called 'alarm clock headache'. More details are provided in chapter 13.

CHAPTER 3

REFERRED PAIN, HEADACHES AFTER HEAD INJURY, AND NEURALGIA

PROBLEMS arising from sites other than 'inside the head' may give rise to headaches. Pains from the eyes, ears, nose, sinuses, teeth, jaws and jaw muscles may all be experienced as headaches. This is what 'referred pain' means – pain arising in one place that is felt somewhere else.

Neuralgia affecting nerves in the head can also give rise to headaches. So, too, can head injuries, although these headaches are usually much less serious than they at first sound.

Eyes

Injuries and infections

Not surprisingly for such a precious organ the eye is very well supplied with nerves. At the merest hint of trouble the eye begins to hurt: a warning that something is wrong. After even quite minor injury or irritation the eye may become very painful, turn red and stream with tears. A headache frequently develops as well. Conjunctivitis (an inflammation of the lining of the eyelids and the covering of the eyeball) and styes (abscesses at the root of eyelashes) may both cause headaches.

Eye strain

Whether eye strain is an important cause of headache is much debated. Certainly many more people think their headaches will be cured by getting spectacles or changing their spectacles than is actually the case.

Problems with focusing, however, seem likely to be responsible for at least some headaches. For example, children who have difficulty reading the blackboard and develop a pain across their forehead find that their headaches disappear once their vision is corrected. Similarly, some people develop headaches after watching a film in a cinema, which requires intense focusing on a screen for a several hours.

If eye strain seems a possible factor in your headaches you should have your eyes tested. If you are advised to get glasses or change the strength of your glasses then take the advice. You may find that the headaches will disappear.

New glasses

Ill- or well-fitting new glasses may cause pain in various muscles of the head (see figure 2), whether from pressure on the nose or temples, or from the frowning involved in keeping them on. People whose glasses are forever slipping down the bridge of their nose should consider plastic lenses, which are lighter than glass.

Glaucoma

Glaucoma is a very important condition which affects one or both eyes and is associated with increased pressure inside the eyeball. It most commonly affects the middle-aged and the elderly. Sometimes there are warning haloes of coloured lights around bright objects. More often, vision gradually fades without pain.

However, acute angle glaucoma is painful – provoking pain in the eye, or above it in the forehead. Because of its effects on vision, glaucoma is a medical emergency. Unfortunately, however, there is often a long delay before anyone connects the pain in the forehead with the eyes. If you experience any of these symptoms, see your doctor immediately. NHS eye tests are free for glaucoma sufferers and for their close relatives aged 40 or over.

Retrobulbar neuritis

In retrobulbar neuritis the optic nerve, at the back of the eye, becomes inflamed. Vision rapidly deteriorates and eye movements may be painful. Medical treatment allows the inflammation to subside and sight returns slowly. The cause is unknown: it may result from a viral infection or an abnormal reaction of the body's immune system.

WARNING

Remember: eyesight is very precious. If you are worried about your eyes see your optician or doctor **quickly**; he or she will direct you to whatever help is necessary.

Ears

External ear

Just as for the eye, injury or inflammation may make the ear painful. A painful external ear – i.e. the ear lobe (*pinna*), the ear hole (*external auditory meatus*) and the eardrum (*tympanic membrane*) – may be due to injured or inflamed skin, which is usually part of a generalised dermatitis. The *external auditory canal*, the passage from the pinna to the eardrum, is lined with skin. A boil in that canal can be very painful.

Middle ear

The middle ear, situated deep to the eardrum, contains three small bones that conduct sound from the eardrum to the inner ear. The middle ear is connected to the back of the throat by the Eustachian tube. Sometimes a difference in pressure may be noticeable – for example, on a train entering a tunnel at high speed or when an aeroplane rapidly changes height. The swallowing mechanism equalises the pressure on both sides of the drum, which is why airlines used to hand out sweets to suck on taking off and landing, and recommend that babies be fed then.

41

If the pressure cannot be equalised, the ear may become painful and a headache develop. One cause of this is *otitis media*, a common complaint in children, which arises when infection tracks from the tonsils up the Eustachian tube into the middle ear. The middle ear then becomes inflamed. The same mechanism applies in *catarrhal otitis* due to sinusitis (see page 44) – thereby causing middle ear pain.

Inner ear

The inner ear deals with hearing and balance. A disturbance of the labyrinth of the inner ear gives rise to vertigo, a sense of rotation similar to the feeling you get after riding on a merry-go-round. Within the inner ear there are a series of semicircular canals, three on each side of the head, which act like spirit levels. They are sited in different planes enabling you to determine whether you are spinning in a horizontal plane, or going up and down in a lift, for example. Some vertigo is 'positional', i.e. moving one's head brings on the giddiness. The importance of vertigo in headache is that if turning your head makes you giddy, you will tend to hold your head and neck rather stiffly. Doing that for very long will bring on pain at the back of the neck, which may well be experienced as a headache. Usually giddiness is short-lived, disappearing completely and quickly. Doctors can prescribe anti-vertigo tablets, which are derived from antihistamines used to combat allergies. As a result tiredness and slow reflexes may be side-effects.

There is another kind of unsteadiness, which is more a lightheadedness than vertigo. Standing to attention or standing for long periods in hot stuffy rooms or train carriages may bring it on, as may hunger and tiredness.

Nose and sinuses

Air is warmed and moistened as it passes up the two nostrils. The sinuses are five cavities in the skull connected by small holes to the main nasal pathway. There are two sinuses in the cheeks (*maxillary sinuses*), two in the forehead (*frontal sinuses*) and one deep behind the bridge of the nose (*sphenoidal sinus*). A lining of

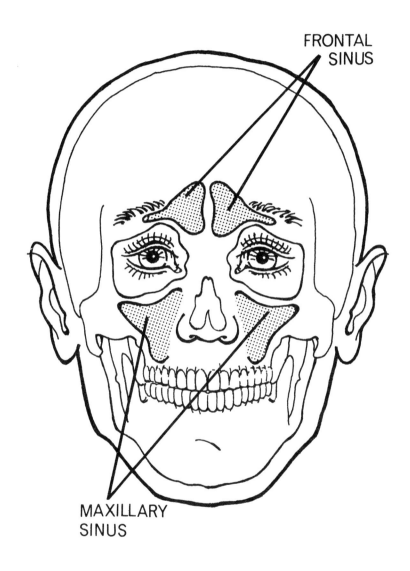

[Figure 3: An outline of the bones of the face, showing the positions of the frontal and maxillary sinuses.]

cells keeps them moist and tiny hairs (*cilia*) on top of the cells move along the moisture (*mucus*) and any debris caught up in it. (These hairs are visible only under the microscope; they look like the top of a wheat field blowing in the wind.)

When one or more of the small openings to the sinuses is blocked, for example during a cold, secretions or air accumulate and become trapped, which can be painful. Inhaling cold air or relieving the pressure inside the sinuses by any of the ways listed below can relieve the pain.

Figure 3 shows that sinus pain can occur on either side of the forehead if the frontal sinuses are inflamed or in either cheek (between the eyes and the upper jaw) if the maxillary sinuses are involved.

Sinusitis, an inflammation of this lining, can become chronic. If this happens, an intermittent discharge of thick green, yellow or clear mucus will trickle down the back of the throat. This will be more noticeable when secretions have accumulated – for example, during the night.

Doctors differ over whether chronic (long-standing) sinusitis can cause headaches, but there is little doubt that acute (of recent onset) sinusitis can.

What can be done?

- Menthol or eucalyptus inhalants. Use these to clear your nose if it is blocked. Keep to the instructions on the bottle: add the required amount of mixture to hot water in a bowl and then inhale. A towel over the head helps to concentrate the steam and the vapours. If that relieves your headache, blocked sinuses are at least contributing to your headache problems even if they are not the sole cause.
- Nasal decongestants. These constrict the lining of the nose relieving the blocked feeling and allowing you to breathe more freely. They should be used for only a few days (in case the lining of the nose becomes irritated), unless otherwise advised by your doctor. If these measures don't relieve your sinus pain, you should consult your doctor. You may need a short course of antibiotics to clear the infection or, in some cases, to have the sinuses washed out.

An injury to the nose can deflect the nasal septum (the cartilage that separates the two sides of the nose), which leads to an obvious deformity on the outside, and obstructs the nasal passages inside. Commonly seen in boxers, this can make nose breathing impossible or produce a local obstruction, so giving rise to sinusitis. In some cases surgery is required.

Less commonly, people complain of a feeling of pressure on the bridge of the nose. So far the cause of this is unknown: it may be due to the small muscles that move the side of the nose becoming contracted and painful.

Teeth, jaws and chewing muscles

Teeth

Localising a painful tooth is usually easy, but occasionally the pain is 'referred', that is, it feels as if it is coming from somewhere else. Pain may be felt in front of, or behind, the affected tooth or further away in the jaw. Less often, the pain is felt in a completely different place – the pain coming from the temple may come from an inflamed tooth in the lower jaw. (This can make life very difficult for the dentist.) Impacted wisdom teeth are a common cause of headaches of this type.

Jaws

If you feel just in front of your ears or put your fingers inside your ears while opening and closing your mouth then you will feel the jaw joints (*temporomandibular joints*) moving. Often the joint creaks or grates, which is sometimes painful. People who grind their teeth at night may wake with painful chewing muscles.

The muscles that open and close the jaw (the masseters and the temporalis muscles in figure 2) are frequently painful. These muscles align the jaw and when the jaw is out of alignment extra stresses are thrown on to them.

What can be done?

- In the first place consult your dentist, who may want to refer you to an oral surgeon or an orthodontist.

Headaches after head injury

It is worth remembering at this point just how well the brain is protected. The skull comprises two layers of thick bone separated by bone marrow – a spongy material that acts like a further shock absorber. So successful is this form of protection that is has been copied by makers of headgear for motor racing and horse-riding.

Concussion means that the brain has been shaken up and the person rendered unconscious for a matter of seconds or minutes; he or she then comes round and is perfectly all right, but might remain mildly confused for a few minutes. Concussion implies unconsciousness: most people referred for consultation have been dazed rather than concussed.

Another important point is that, if the skull is fractured, the underlying brain often remains uninjured. It is exactly like a crash helmet being dented, but the person underneath remaining perfectly healthy. A fractured skull, surprisingly, is often less serious a problem – if you are going to have a head injury – than concussion.

Most head injuries do not damage the brain but do give rise to a host of fears. A further common anxiety is that further trouble may develop after the injury. This, too, is not the case.

The commonest headache after the head injury is due to anxiety or tension and has the characteristics described under tension headache, namely, a sensation of continuous pressure.

However, there is a state after head injury in which the person is nervous, has difficulty in going to sleep, may over-breathe (hyperventilate) and tend to feel giddy. That person needs a careful neurological examination and reassurance that there is nothing amiss in the head or brain.

There is an important rider: if someone has been unconscious for a minute or longer, these comments do not apply. Medical advice is needed in such cases.

What can be done?

If you can clearly recall the circumstances of the head injury and if a skull X-ray taken at the time (or later) was normal, there is unlikely to be anything seriously wrong with the brain. Serious problems are similarly rare after head injuries followed by short periods of unconsciousness and amnesia (lack of recall) lasting for 5 to 10 minutes after the head injury.

SYMPTOMS

- Unconsciousness – the patient is unaware of external circumstances; incapable of responding to sensory stimuli; the patient cannot be roused (hence not sleep)
- Coma – a state of profound unconsciousness, from which the sufferer cannot be raised even by stimulation
- Concussion – paralysis of the functions of the brain as an immediate consequence of a blow to the head; has a strong tendency to a spontaneous recovery
- Stupor – degree of altered consciousness in which the patient responds to simple, but not complex, commands or stimuli
- Daze – stupefaction or bewilderment, though remaining conscious
- Fainting – loss of consciousness due to fall in blood pressure which may occur at the sight of blood, or standing to attention, as in soldiers on parade.

Neuralgia

Shingles and post-shingles pain

Zoster*, the shingles virus (which is the same as the chickenpox virus), has a predilection for the head and upper trunk, involving a single nerve on one side only. Usually the forehead is affected.

With shingles there may be pain a few days before an eruption of chickenpox-like blisters appears. Then the blisters appear in the distribution of the affected nerve. When this clears, small scars may remain. For some time after the eruption has gone

* Zoster is the name of the virus; herpes (blisters) is the skin eruption, which can be due to a number of viruses.

there may be pain in the area supplied by the nerve – post-herpetic neuralgia. Not all attacks of shingles are followed by post-herpetic neuralgia – it is, however, more likely the older you are. Because shingles and chickenpox are caused by the same virus, someone with shingles can give a child chickenpox and vice versa.

What can be done?

- The drug acyclovir is an antiviral drug which acts against viruses and has to be prescribed by a doctor. It may be useful if given early in the attack. Drugs are also available for the treatment of post-herpetic neuralgia; the most common one being used at present is carbamazepine which dampens irritated nerve fibres. It is also highly effective in trigeminal neuralgia (see below).

Trigeminal neuralgia

This is another sort of neuralgia affecting the face. It produces a sudden pain 'like an electric shock' that usually begins in one spot in the cheek, lip or lower part of the face. The pain shoots in one direction, similar to the pain experienced when a dentist touches a nerve in an exposed bit of dentine. The sudden jab is usually followed by an afterglow of dull pain that lasts maybe a minute. Touching or moving the affected part of the face will bring on an attack.

The list of triggers includes:
- chewing
- washing
- shaving
- speaking
- a cold wind blowing on the face.

The cause of trigeminal neuralgia is not known.

What can be done?

- A drug called carbamazepine, available on prescription, often helps. Sometimes surgery is necessary.

CHAPTER 4

SOME SERIOUS BUT RARE CAUSES OF HEADACHES

THE HEADACHES described in this chapter are not common conditions. For each, early medical assistance is essential. It is worth pointing out that the headache will rarely be the only symptom and that the severity of a headache is a poor guide to the seriousness of its underlying cause. The most painful headaches are migraine and cluster headaches – not the causes listed here.

Tumours

Contrary to popular belief, a headache is not a very prominent symptom of a brain tumour: mostly there are other symptoms caused by the tumour pressing on part of the brain and affecting its function. For example, a tumour in the front of the brain may produce personality changes (evident to relatives although not the patients), or lead to a failing memory. Pressing on one side of the brain, a tumour may produce weakness or decreased sensitivity of the opposite side of the body because most brain fibres cross somewhere as they descend to their destination. Tumours at the back of the brain, can interfere with vision, giving rise to a loss of part of the visual field.

If a tumour presses on that portion of the brain underneath the temple (the temporal lobe) and on the left side (in right-handed people), speech and writing difficulties can arise.

Epileptic fits (or convulsions) may result from the tumour acting as a focus of irritation in the brain. (Most people with epileptic fits, however, do not have brain tumours.)

When headaches occur in the presence of a tumour, it is usually because the tumour is interfering with the circulation of fluid bathing the brain (the cerebrospinal fluid). This usually occurs quite late in the process, after other symptoms have developed.

Meningitis

The meninges are three layers of protective membranes covering the brain: an outer hard protective layer (*dura*); a blood vessel layer and a very thin layer (*pia-arachnoid*). Inflammation of these tissues is known as meningitis.

Meningitis may be due to:

- viruses
- bacteria
- blood.

Not all cases of meningitis, however, are equally serious – for example, children with mumps often have meningitis as part of their illness, which usually clears up without any lasting ill effects. People with mild forms of viral meningitis may feel that they have nothing worse than a bad attack of flu and keep on working.

Meningitis due to a bacterial infection, where germs have circulated in the bloodstream and reached the brain, is another matter – it requires prompt medical attention and treatment with antibiotics. Meningococcal meningitis is often associated with a skin rash, but other bacteria like the pneumococcus can cause the same dangerous clinical condition. Provided the bacteria are identified quickly and treatment with the right antibiotic is started early enough, patients usually do very well.

When blood vessels on the surface of the brain rupture (usually after severe head injury), the red cells released act as irritants to the meninges and a 'chemical' meningitis develops, requiring immediate medical treatment.

Aneurysms and subarachnoid haemorrhage

Sometimes the walls of arteries supplying the brain can dilate and these dilated segments (known as aneurysms) may rupture, producing a bleed called a subarachnoid haemorrhage. This may happen when a person suffers from high blood pressure.

A sudden, very intense headache follows. Individuals say it feels like being struck down by a hammer blow. This is a medical emergency and requires urgent admission to hospital.

Subdural haematoma

Just as blood vessels in the skin or eye may leak spontaneously, giving rise to a bruise, so too may the blood vessels on the surface of the brain. This may also follow minor injury to the head, particularly in the elderly. The result is a surface blood clot (subdural haematoma). If the clot is large enough it can produce a steadily worsening headache, gradually deteriorating or causing oscillating levels of consciousness and other signs similar to those of a brain tumour. Surgery may be needed to remove the clot although some resolve themselves.

Obstructive hydrocephalus

The brain is bathed in cerebrospinal fluid, and if its circulation is blocked pressure may build up, sometimes resulting in a headache. Blockages usually follow inflammation – either from infection or from blood leaking into the cerebrospinal fluid. This problem can be treated by inserting a tube connecting the cavities of the brain to the lining of the abdominal wall or to one of the veins that enters the heart. Interestingly, this treatment was suggested by an engineer whose child had congenital hydrocephalus: the device, the Spitz-Holter valve, bears the names of the father and the surgeon.

Benign intracranial hypertension

In this condition headaches are caused by increased pressure inside the head. Its cause is unknown, but young, overweight women are most commonly affected. In some cases it seems related to taking the oral contraceptive pill or to steroids. The condition may lead to blindness if the pressure stays too high for too long.

It may be necessary for the person to lose weight or stop taking the offending tablets (medical advice should be sought first). Specialist help is usually needed from a neurologist or neurosurgeon.

High blood pressure

For blood pressure to cause a headache it has to be extremely high – high enough to make the brain swell, which is very unusual. This happens when raised blood pressure increases rapidly to enter a 'malignant' phase, or during pregnancy as part of eclampsia. Both are medical emergencies, requiring speedy hospital admission. Being told that they have high blood pressure makes some people anxious, and the resulting anxiety can cause tension headaches (see page 31), which are then mistakenly ascribed to high blood pressure. Increases in blood pressure (hypertension) can be controlled by hypotensive drugs.

Brain oedema

Brain oedema, a very rare condition, occurs when the brain swells, and is usually associated with some disturbance of metabolism. Cortisone is one cause, but this is very rare. However, intoxication with lead or tin does occur in children and that can give rise to headache resulting from brain oedema.

Giant cell arteritis

This rare cause of headache virtually never affects anyone under 55. In giant cell 'arteritis' (inflammation of artery walls), the walls become infiltrated by 'giant cells' and other inflammatory cells, visible only under the microscope. The inflamed arteries become painful and swollen. Typically affected are the arteries lying over the temporalis muscles (see page 33), hence the condition is often called temporal arteritis. Other superficial and deeper arteries of the head may also be involved.

People with giant cell arteritis complain of severe headaches that may prevent them lying on the affected area and even combing and brushing their hair. These localised manifestations are part of a generalised illness which gives rise to fever, poor appetite, weight loss and muscle pains.

For a diagnosis to be made, a small segment of an affected artery may need to be biopsied and checked for the characteristic appearance of giant cell arteritis under the microscope. This is usually done under a local anaesthetic.

The symptoms respond dramatically to steroids which may have to be continued for many months until the inflammation settles down. Left untreated, the vessels supplying the eye may become affected, resulting in blindness. To check the progress of the disease, regular blood tests, including measuring the erythrocyte sedimentation rate (the rate of aggregation of red blood cells), are performed.

BLOOD PRESSURE

Blood pressure is measured by two values and is expressed as a systolic figure over a diastolic figure. Systolic is the higher pressure of the two and represents the reading during the heartbeat (contraction of the heart) when blood is pumped into the aorta. Diastolic is the lower reading and represents the stage when the ventricles in the heart relax between beats.

A standard reading is 120/80 but up to 140/90 is normal and many people are perfectly well with a blood pressure of 100/60. 'Malignant hypertension' is usually associated with a blood pressure above 200/150 and is characterised by brain swelling (oedema).

PART 2

COPING WITH HEADACHES

CHAPTER 5

COPING ON YOUR OWN

IF YOU do suffer from headaches, the first person to turn to is yourself. Although there are drugs (see below), doctors (see chapter 6) and a variety of complementary therapies which may work by helping you avoid the trigger factors causing headaches and/or help lessen the pain once a headache has started, the onus is on the individual to take responsibility for seeking the best advice available. This chapter is devoted to finding out what you can do for yourself, without recourse to experts.

Before you can do much, though, it is important to have some idea of what is causing your headache. With so many different possibilities, from eating ice-cream to tension, it is not surprising that there is no one common treatment that works for all headaches. Treatments vary according to root cause: if you can discover what is provoking your headaches then you have a good chance of avoiding them.

PAIN

Pain, wherever it comes from, is the body's way of saying that something is wrong. Headaches are no different. The message is that headaches are the end result of an underlying problem; the challenge is to discover what that is.

The first four chapters of this book have given an idea of the range of possible underlying causes of headaches, most of them not serious. Listed in chapter 4 are the few that are. Trying to manage these yourself would be not only useless but dangerous. These headaches make up only a very small proportion of all the headaches from which people suffer.

Establishing the facts

What can you do if after reading this far you are still no nearer an understanding of why you get your headaches? You may need to ask yourself the following questions concerning your headaches:

- How long have I been getting them?
- Did they follow any change in my life?
- Does anything seem to bring them on?
- Is there anything special about the circumstances in which they develop, for example, the time of day, day of the week, or before a particular event?
- What makes them better? Worse?
- What do they stop me from doing? Is it something I miss or is it something I secretly dread?

Some pattern may emerge from this self-interrogation to give you a lead. Talk to members of your family or someone else who knows you and your headaches well. Can they shed any light on the problem? Often it takes someone else to recognise when you are tense or anxious or under a lot of pressure. (And if someone suggests you are, take him or her seriously; anxious people often have great difficulty in believing that anything is wrong.) As more headaches are caused by stress than anything else you should think quite hard whether this could be an important factor.

Keeping a diary

If there are still no clues, keep a headache diary for a few weeks.
- Note the time of day and the day of the week that headaches occur and for how long they last.
- What is their relationship, if any, to meals? Does eating make them better? Do they seem to follow particular foods or drink?
- Do you take any tablets for your headache? If so, make a note

of the type, how effective they are and how quickly they act, and how long the improvement lasts.

- Are they worse during particularly stressful periods or after physical exercise?
- Women should record their menstruation. Do the headaches have any relationship to menstruation?

From just a few weeks of records a pattern may emerge. If you decide you then need to consult a doctor about your headaches, such a headache diary will be very useful.

Can you identify a trigger?

Obviously, if you have found something that seems to trigger your headaches then you should do your best to avoid it. But this may be a counsel of perfection: for working mothers, for instance, the pressures of juggling a career and a family may cause unavoidable stress, thereby resulting in headaches.

Stress

If you think that stress may be inducing your headaches, there are several things you can do.
- Investigate any local classes offering yoga or meditation or other relaxation techniques. Make contact with any local self-help group that might offer you support and assistance. The British Wheel of Yoga is the co-ordinating body in England and Wales. See the address on page 175 for details of where to ring for advice on local groups in your area.
- Many complementary therapies aim to reduce stress. The most well-known therapies – acupuncture, the Alexander Technique, aromatherapy and yoga – are described in the appendix.
- If you aren't fit, consider getting fit, *gradually*. What you should do to get fit depends very much on your age and your general level of health. Long walks and swimming should be within just about everybody's reach. How about jogging, cycling or aerobics classes. People who are fit not only feel healthy but seem better at shaking off the stresses and strains that come everybody's way.

- Try progressive relaxation exercises. If you want to practise relaxation, you should allow at least a quarter of an hour a day and try to follow the same sequence every time.

Relaxing surroundings are helpful but not essential. It is best (at least at first) to choose a quiet, dimly-lit room where you can be warm and comfortable and not subject to distractions. Relaxation should be enjoyable, otherwise it will not work. Begin by taking off your shoes and loosening any tight clothing, especially at the neck and waist. Adopt a relaxed posture: the easiest is probably lying down.

1. Lie down on a carpeted floor, or a bed – provided it is not too soft. All parts of your body should be supported comfortably. Lie with your arms and legs a little apart. It is better to do without a pillow.

2. Tense and relax every part of your body in turn, starting either with hands and arms, then head and down through the trunk to the legs, or starting with the feet and legs and working up through the body.

3. If you begin with the hands and arms, you should first clench the fists, which also entails clenching the forearm muscles. Hold this for a little while, perhaps ten seconds, and feel the tension; then let go and feel the difference – a sensation of welcome release. Then hold the hands (fists clenched) against the shoulders so as to tense the upper arms, feel the tension, and then let go.

4. Hold the neck taut with the chin pressed in, then relaxed, followed by the different facial muscles – forehead (frown and relax), eyebrows (raise up then release), eyes, mouth (purse up and release), jaw (thrust forward and release), then the shoulders (hunch up then let go), stomach, buttocks, thighs, legs and feet. Each time you should consciously feel the tension before you let go.

5. After tensing and relaxing each muscle group in turn, you should feel relaxed all over. Instead of thinking of yourself in parts, be aware of the whole body and if you feel any remaining tension anywhere, try to release it – if necessary by first deliberately tensing the affected muscles and then letting go.

6. Allow five to ten minutes at the end in which to enjoy your relaxed state. You should be breathing quietly, with slow and gentle breaths. You may want to imagine a peaceful scene, for instance lying peacefully by the side of a blue lake, with green grass and trees, the song of the birds, the warmth of the sun, your body warm, heavy and relaxed. Choose your own imagined scene – whatever you like best.

7. When you are ready to get up, first have a good stretch, then either sit up very slowly or turn over (on to your side first into what is called 'the recovery position'), then get up.

Your aim should be to carry over your relaxed state into whatever activity follows your period of relaxation.

Although it is easier to practise relaxation while lying down, sitting is also all right. You can practise in an armchair – and in time you should be able to relax even in an office chair or on a bus or in the driver's seat of a parked car or wherever you happen to be.

Staying relaxed

Once the technique of relaxation has been learned, it should be possible to relax without first tensing all the muscles and it should be easy to detect any areas of tension and quickly release it in these areas.

Throughout the day, get into the habit of checking whether you are tensing any muscles unnecessarily. If you are, you are not only wasting energy and effort but could well bring on headache, neckache and backache.

If your face is tensed and mouth turned downward, relax it and consciously force the corners of your lips upwards into a smile. It may be mechanical, but it helps you to feel less dejected or stressed.

Treating the symptoms

So far in this book headaches have been regarded as symptoms and the search has been on to track down their cause. What is used to justify this is the belief that if causes can be removed then the headaches may go. But sometimes little or nothing can be done about the cause – even when the trigger has been identified. So what are the ways in which you can dispel a headache by using medication?

Pain relievers

Pain relievers (or analgesics) are very good at dulling the pain. If you decide to use them (rather than some of the complementary methods described in the appendix), take them early in the course of the headache. There are two reasons for this.

The first is that if you wait too long – thinking that your headache might go of its own accord – then it may build up to such an intensity that ordinary pain relievers won't work. The second reason is that nausea or sickness may stop the tablets being absorbed and therefore the drugs become less effective or ineffective. Analgesics do not cure a headache, they only relieve the pain for three to four hours.

If you can't stop the headaches coming on, you can do your best to stop them getting worse. This may mean carying your pain relievers with you. But which preparation? In terms of their effects on pain there is not much to choose between aspirin, paracetamol and codeine either on their own or in combination with each other and with caffeine.

What you can be sure of is that any combination sold under a trade name will be more expensive than a single drug sold under its proprietary name. Some people may find that one drug or combination of drugs works better for them – if so, they should certainly stick to it. But there is no scientific evidence that one preparation is better than another when tested on large numbers of people with headaches. Soluble (or dispersible) formulations may enter the blood system more quickly than tablets, and some experts argue that they also offer some form of protection against gastro-intestinal irritation.

Over-the-counter medication

The following preparations are available over the counter to help relieve the pain of headaches. They can also help with migraine. See also page 120 for further details of over-the-counter and prescription drugs used to treat headaches and migraine. It is always advisable to consult a pharmacist or your GP before using any drugs.

Always take tablets and capsules with several swallows of a drink – at least half a cup – while standing or sitting up. Do not take your medicine lying down – tablets may stick in your gullet and injure it.

Aspirin

Aspirin has anti-inflammatory properties and is an antipyretic (reduces fever). It is also a gastric irritant and may increase the risk of bleeding from the stomach in those with a history of indigestion or ulcers. Other groups of people who should avoid aspirin include people taking anti-coagulants (blood thinners for certain heart conditions), asthmatics, those who suffer from allergic reactions and women during pregnancy. If, while taking aspirin, your motions become black and tarry, you should immediately stop taking the tablets and seek medical help. The Committee on the Safety of Medicines (CSM) has recommended that aspirin should not be given to children under 12 because of the links with Reye's syndrome. Recommended dose: 300-900mg (1-3 tablets) every four to six hours (daily maximum 4g).

Paracetamol

Paracetamol has none of the side-effects ascribed to aspirin, has no anti-inflammatory properties and is less of an irritant than aspirin. Overdosage, however, is potentially very dangerous, resulting in liver damage, which may go undetected for four to six days. Otherwise, side-effects are very rare. Recommended dose: 500mg-1g (1-2 tablets) every four to six hours. Do not take at intervals of less than four hours (daily maximum 4g).

Ibuprofen

Like aspirin, ibuprofen is an anti-inflammatory drug; unlike aspirin it is not associated with Reye's syndrome. It is not recommended for people who are allergic to aspirin, or asthmatics. Recommended dose: up to 1.8g daily in divided doses.

Caffeine

Caffeine is often included in pain-reliever combinations to give a feeling of alertness. It may also enhance the pain-relieving properties of aspirin or paracetamol.

Codeine

Codeine is an opioid analgesic and is sold over the counter only in combination with aspirin or paracetamol. There are constipating effects after long-term use.

You should remember that all drugs have unpleasant side-effects in some people, and simple pain relievers, available over the counter without prescription, are no exception. So it is always necessary to read the label before taking any preparation.

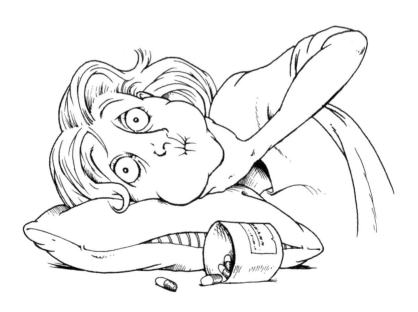

[Figure 4: 'Do not take your medicine lying down.']

When to visit your doctor?

- When you develop a new kind of headache, a new pattern of headaches, or when there is something unusual about the pain.
- When a headache begins suddenly, especially if associated with neck stiffness, vomiting or a rash.
- When a headache is associated with neck stiffness and fever.
- When the pain is too severe to be relieved by ordinary pain relievers.
- When headaches become increasingly frequent or when their frequency interferes with work, social life or leisure interests.
- If the headache attacks increase in duration or intensity.
- If other disturbances accompany the headache, for example:
  - your sight or balance is affected
  - you feel faint or lose consciousness during attacks
  - you are losing your appetite or experiencing weight loss
  - you develop a weakness or numbness on one side of your body or face
  - your speech, memory or vision is affected.
- If the headaches are making you depressed.
- When the headaches have begun soon after you have started new medication.
- When the headaches are beginning to worry you or other members of your family.

CHAPTER **6**

COPING WITH MEDICAL HELP

DECIDING to take their medical problem to a doctor makes most people anxious – even if only slightly. There is so much to be worried about. Some people are frightened of looking silly, bothering the doctor with what he or she will regard as a minor problem. Others fear that medicine will have nothing to offer them. Most unpleasant of all would be having their worst suspicions confirmed. As has already been stated this last outcome is very unlikely – serious underlying causes account for only a very small number of all the headaches suffered. Some symptoms, listed on page 65, should make you consult your doctor without delay.

Which doctor?

In Britain, your first port of call will be your general practitioner. Mostly he or she will come to a decision that regardless of how incapacitating your headaches are, there is nothing sinister going on. Your doctor will then suggest a course of action.

If your general practitioner is not sure about what is causing your headaches or if what has been recommended has not helped, you may be referred to a specialist. This will usually be a neurologist, although it could be a rheumatologist, or an ear, nose and throat or eye specialist.

To become a consultant in Britain, doctors train in a speciality for six to eight years after three years of general medical and surgical experience. They may have devoted a few years to research as well.

By the time they see you there is a 99.9 per cent chance that they will have come across a case like yours before. People either ask or want to ask, 'Have you ever seen a case like mine before?', thinking that they are unique. The answer is: 'Yes, you are unique, but your disease is not'. And, unlike many problems for which a medical opinion is sought, with headaches, you can be reasonably sure that your doctor knows what you're talking about: as 95 to 98 per cent of the population suffer from headaches then so too will 95 to 98 per cent of doctors.

What to expect from your doctor

Before beginning treatment doctors first try to diagnose what is wrong. To do this they rely on three separate elements. The first is the *history* of the complaint, which is obtained by listening and putting questions to the person and his or her relatives. The second is what is found on *examination*, which may be limited in the case of headaches to just the head or may take in the whole body. The third (and only in a few cases) is what is provided by special *investigations*.

How much these three contribute to the making of a diagnosis varies according to the condition. Skin conditions, such as eczema and psoriasis, may be diagnosed just by examining the patient, while blood disorders can be diagnosed only after laboratory tests have been performed.

Medical history

Doctors expect to diagnose the cause of a headache almost entirely from a person's medical history. So be prepared for a lot of talking, not much examination and few special tests. Questions that your doctor may ask you include:

- When did the headaches start?
- How often do they occur?
- How long do they last?
- What precedes them?
- What brings them on?

- Where do the headaches start?
- Does the pain move during an attack?
- Is the pain superficial or deep?
- Does anything make the headache worse (for example, coughing, straining or bending down)?
- What makes them better?
- What is the pain like?★
- How severe is it?
- Is it associated with anything else (such as nausea or a dislike of bright lights)?
- Does any other member of your family have headaches?
- What sort of an effect do headaches have on your life?
- What have you already tried for the headaches and what effect did this have?
- What do you think is causing the pain?
- Why have you decided to seek help now?
- What are you worried about?

Few doctors will ask you *all* these questions, but it might be helpful to decide beforehand how you would answer each of them. The better quality information you provide, the more chance the doctor has of making the right diagnosis and suggesting effective treatment.

Expect other questions about your general health, and perhaps about your nervous system as well. Your doctor may ask about your senses of smell, taste, sight and hearing, and your speech, balance, memory, concentration, sleeping and mood. Many of the questions you will be asked may seem to have nothing whatsoever to do with your headaches and be time wasting. But they are important.

Medical examination

Similarly with your physical examination. You may be asked to undress to your underclothes and the extent of examination may

---

★ This may be difficult to answer and further questions may be asked, such as, 'Is it aching, burning, gripping, throbbing, pressing, turning, a discomfort, or just an awareness?' or 'What would you do to someone else to reproduce your symptoms – stick a knife or needle into the skin, apply pressure, or hammer the area?'.

once again seem bizarre. Why, for instance, is the doctor so interested in your feet when you went complaining of a headache?

For the consultation to work there has to be trust on both sides. You should be able to trust your doctor to ask the appropriate questions, examine you properly and request the right tests. Similarly, your doctor should be able to trust you to answer his questions to the best of your ability. If you have kept a headache diary (see page 58) it may prove to be invaluable.

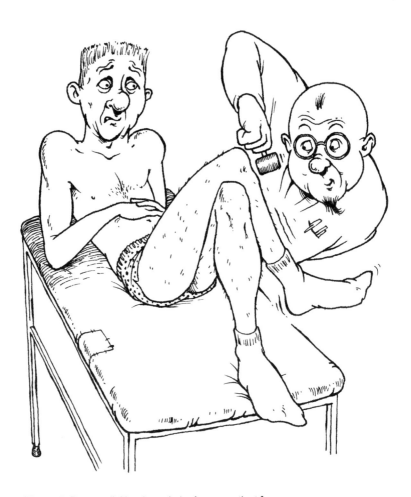

[Figure 5: Doctor eliciting knee jerks from a patient.]

Investigations

Doctors expect the results of most investigations performed in people who have been suffering from headaches for a long time to be normal and will request few tests. They may arrange:

- blood tests.
- X-rays – of your sinuses (see page 44) if sinusitis is suspected or of your neck if arthritis is suspected. (Skull X-rays are rarely requested: they are very useful for deciding whether you have fractured your skull but, in the absence of injury, they are of little value in identifying the cause of headaches.)
- computerised tomography (CT or CAT scan). Multiple X-ray views of the brain are taken and a computer produces a series of detailed images of the brain as if it had been sliced very thinly. For this the person's head is introduced into a scanner and he/she is asked to lie very still for about 20 to 30 minutes. An injection of dye may be given into the arm, which is sometimes followed by an unpleasant, hot sensation, which is fortunately shortlived.
- arteriography. In this test dye is injected into neck arteries and a series of X-rays of the head is taken. The arteries supply the brain, the dye reveals their distribution there, which is usually abnormal if the headache has a serious underlying cause. Because the procedure is noisy and unpleasant it is usually performed under a general anaesthetic. But with the wider availability of CT scans fewer arteriograms are now performed.
- lumbar puncture. This may be performed in cases where headaches are of relatively sudden onset and either meningitis or a bleeding blood vessel is suspected. In this test the person lies on one side and a needle is introduced between the vertebrae of the lower back. A specimen of cerebrospinal fluid (which bathes the spinal cord and the brain) is removed and analysed for the presence of blood, bacteria and other constituents like sugar and protein.
- arterial biopsy. If cranial arteritis is suspected, then a small specimen of one of the superficial arteries of the forehead or scalp is sometimes excised and examined under a microscope.

After the diagnosis is made

Most people with headaches who consult their doctor do so for reassurance that 'nothing is wrong' – i.e. there is no brain tumour or blood vessel about to burst. Fortunately, in most cases this can be given, either at the first consultation or after investigations have been performed.

What follows reassurance? A diagnosis suggests a course of action. If trigger factors have been identified, avoiding these will be recommended, for example, more sleep, no red wine before periods, or fewer missed meals.

Unfortunately, many people seem predisposed to headaches, with trigger factors either hidden or beyond their control. Even if it is not possible to cure their headaches then some relief can usually be given so that attacks become less frequent or more manageable, or both.

And, finally, drugs have an important place in the treatment of longstanding, troublesome headaches when other techniques have been tried and have failed.

PART 3

MIGRAINES

CHAPTER 7

WHAT IS A MIGRAINE ATTACK?

SOME PEOPLE suspect that migraine is a fancy name for headache; this is not so. A migraine, with its specific symptoms that occur before, during and after attacks, differs profoundly from other headaches.

A TYPICAL MIGRAINE ATTACK

You enter her bedroom, which is very quiet and dark. The curtains are drawn – she dislikes light and noise and is trying to avoid these as much as possible. Because moving her head increases the pain, she lies still in bed. She looks drawn and pale – 'as white as a sheet' or 'as pale as a ghost'. The room is warm: feeling cold she is trying to get warmer. The room smells because she has been vomiting; a bowl is beside the bed. Sitting up to vomit she holds her head since vomiting accentuates her deep-seated throbbing headache.

Pain and nausea make her feel hot and cold alternately, and after vomiting several times she sweats. The vomiting and lack of food leave her feeling weak. The smell of cooking or even perfume may be very unpleasant, increasing the nausea.

Even the vibration of footsteps can increase the pain. Holding her head may bring a little comfort, but real, lasting improvement comes only from sleeping, which occurs after several hours of intense pain.

What is migraine?

There is no universally accepted definition of migraine. The *Concise Oxford Dictionary* gives the following description: 'recurrent throbbing headache that usually affects one side of the head, often accompanied by nausea and disturbance of vision.'

A fuller definition of migraine is 'an episodic headache that comes at intervals lasting between two and 72 hours with total freedom between attacks, which must be accompanied by visual or gastro-intestinal disturbances or both. The visual symptoms may occur as an aura before the headache or as a dislike of light during the headache. The gastro-intestinal upset consists of nausea and vomiting; if there are no visual disturbances then vomiting must feature in some of the attacks.'

If it weren't so unpleasant a migraine attack could be compared to a symphony of five movements.

The five stages of a migraine are (in order):

- premonitory symptoms
- aura
- headache and other symptoms
- resolution of a migraine attack
- migraine postdromes or 'hangover'.

Each of the first three stages may occur in isolation. The five stages of an attack are described in detail below.

Premonitory symptoms

Migraine sufferers may be aware of an impending attack of migraine in the 24 hours before it starts. The symptoms can be subtle and recalled only in retrospect. Sometimes they are more noticeable to those who live or work with the sufferer.

Non-medical writers have provided good descriptions of this stage. For instance, George Eliot felt 'dangerously well before an attack'; Edith, in Anita Brookner's *Hotel du Lac*, saw everything as very bright on Friday evening, then woke the next morning with a severe headache. Lady Conway (a patient in Dr Thomas Willis' *Casebook*, dated 1683) would eat her supper with a greedy appetite and then her 'pain would almost certainly follow the next morning'.

Between one and two of every three migraine sufferers experience some form of warning of an impending attack. For some the warnings are not always followed by headaches. The commonest premonitory symptoms are described below:

Variation in mood
Sufferers may feel 'high' or 'low'. Some may become witty or extroverted or experience 'a Napoleonic feeling', that is, they think they can conquer the world. One woman described herself as 'all systems go, on top of the world', while another felt that she could do all the spring-cleaning in a day. One sufferer's mother described her daughter as 'ebullient and jocular'.

On the other hand some people feel low and tense, depressed

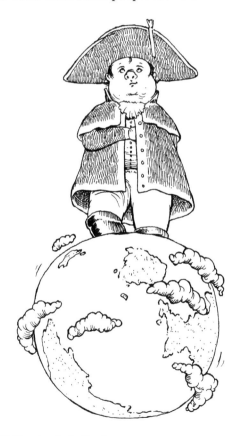

[Figure 6: 'A Napoleonic feeling.']

and quiet before an attack. One described himself as feeling like a caged animal. A few become irritable and indecisive.

Tiredness, yawning and altered speech

Sufferers may yawn or sigh deeply without feeling tired; others experience both symptoms. One sufferer described himself as 'fuzzy and muddle-headed', another as 'mentally hazy and clumsy'. Some people may have difficulty in finding the right word, which contributes to their general feeling of muddle-headedness.

Stomach symptoms

Hunger, particularly the desire for sweet foods or carbohydrates like bread, biscuits or toast, is common. Quite a few sufferers have a craving for chocolate. It may be that instead of chocolate provoking an attack of migraine (as commonly believed) the desire for this form of nourishment is a sign that the attack has already begun. These premonitory symptoms are reminiscent of the cravings typical of pregnancy.

Fluid retention

Some sufferers retain fluid. This is more likely in women with premenstrual migraine, who may feel bloated and swollen before their period. Others on the day before an attack may notice that they pass more urine.

Other symptoms

Sometimes, before an attack of migraine, people experience muscular pains or heaviness, particularly in the back of the neck and in the limbs. Even in this early phase a few may dread light and noise. Because their skin feels irritable they may not want to be touched. Occasionally, sufferers have diarrhoea or open their bowels more frequently before the attacks begin.

These early symptoms resemble those that occur during an attack. They may persist, becoming worse as the headache develops or even last until the headache has disappeared.

Auras

These symptoms can be traced to temporary dysfunction of parts of the brain and are thought to be due to reduced blood flow there. (For a fuller discussion of theories of migraine see chapter 10.) The particular symptoms depend on which part of the brain is receiving too little blood for its needs.

Auras usually develop gradually over a period of 5 to 20 minutes and last less than an hour. A headache usually follows within an hour.

Visual disturbances

These are the 'classical' auras of migraine and are believed to arise from reduced blood flow to the occipital lobes, the specialised part at the back of the brain concerned with vision.

Auras may comprise flashing lights or an arc of light. More typically they are angular – imagine a jagged rainbow with silvery colours. The visual disturbance may start in one corner of the eye as a flickering light and then move across the field of vision, sometimes stopping halfway. In some people the aura starts in the centre like a star, which then expands outwards. Tunnel vision can occur; for example, one musician who started a migraine attack during a performance found he could read just the few bars of the score he was playing.

Another visual disturbance is a blind spot, which can enlarge to blot out the whole field of vision. Or it can be a sudden blacking out, or greying out, of the whole visual field. Some auras entail the (temporary) loss of half of the field of vision: nothing can be seen to the right (or left) with either eye.

These symptoms usually arise slowly: someone driving a car, for example, would have enough time to pull over and stop. The symptoms usually disappear after 10 to 20 minutes.

Another typical visual disturbance is an outline like the top of a castle, which explains the use of the term 'fortification spectra'. Sometimes an object is outlined in bright lights. These visual disturbances may be very worrying; initially many people believe that they are going blind. These auras are usually followed by headache, though this is not always the case.

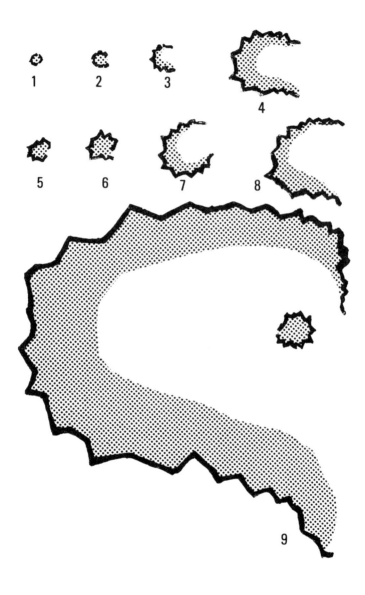

[Figure 7: Dr Hubert Airy's drawing of his own visual disturbances drawn at timed intervals.]

CASE HISTORY

A doctor described how, while driving to work, the number plate of the car in front of him disappeared, being replaced by a wall of greyness. Within a minute, he could see the number plate (implying that his central vision had returned), but then the blank area spread as a circle right to the edge of his visual field – the whole process took exactly 19 minutes. Each time he subsequently experienced these disturbances his timings of them showed the effect to take *exactly* 19 minutes.

Such visual patterns are highly repetitive. There is a famous series of drawings made by Dr Hubert Airy of his own visual auras. These accompanied his description of a 'transient hemiopsia' read by his father, the Astronomer Royal, to the Royal Society in 1870.

The patterns are amazingly similar to those drawn today by migraine sufferers in the competitions run by the British Migraine Association. In these, members of the association are asked to draw what migraine represents or how it looks to them. Many draw visual auras and their patterns are surprisingly similar, with the zigzags and jagged edges described above turning up regularly.

Other disturbances

Auras need not be visual. Other symptoms may occur in the hour before the headache: pins and needles or numbness spreading up an arm to the face, tingling around the mouth, or even weakness of one side of the body. Occasionally the power of speech is lost.

When migraine affects the basilar artery supplying the brain stem, the aura may also include slurring of speech, giddiness, tinnitus (ringing in the ears), decreased hearing, double vision and unsteadiness. As with visual auras, these abnormalities return to normal as the headache develops.

Rarely, in complicated cases, these symptoms may persist for hours or even days. Double vision, which is short-lived, may follow paralysis of a nerve supplying an eye muscle.

Fear

During the aura, before the headache begins, certain people feel very afraid. There are several reasons: for some, the aura symptoms are very bizarre and may include hallucinations and trance-like states. Not surprisingly, they worry that they may be suffering from mental illness. Others may feel acutely apprehensive about the severity of the headache to come and the resulting incapacity.

Migraine attacks, in general, seem to be associated with a fear of specific forthcoming events, such as social commitments, from which sufferers worry their attacks will keep them. Some people complain that their lives have contracted because their migraine has made them frightened of making arrangements that they may not be able to keep.

Headache, vomiting and photophobia: the 'essence' of a migraine

'The essential feature of migraine is paroxysmal headache . . . and is very seldom absent; next in frequency are nausea and vomiting, then some disturbances of vision.' So wrote Sir William Gowers, a founding father of British neurology, more than a hundred years ago. His description remains true today. Let us look at these symptoms (and a few more less common ones) in detail.

Headache

The pain usually begins slowly, coming on at any time of the day. On the morning of a migraine the sufferer often wakes with discomfort in the head, which increases gradually over several hours. The pain is usually restricted to one side of the head.★

After building up slowly, the discomfort becomes an ache and later a throbbing pain. Often, there is a mixture of the two, so that an ache is present continuously but, when the person walks, say, to the toilet, or gets out of bed to vomit, the pain becomes

★ The word 'migraine' is a shortened version of the Greek *hemicrania* – a headache on one side of the head. However, the pain of a migraine may affect both sides or be felt centrally.

throbbing for a few minutes. Sufferers frequently complain that their head feels as if it is bursting, making them want to clasp it with both hands.

CASE HISTORY

Maybe the 'bursting' sensation is appropriate. More than 50 years ago a nurse who had experienced migraines for some years developed symptoms that made her doctors suspect that she had a brain tumour. When she was operated on, no tumour was found, but in those days the piece of skull which was removed to explore the brain was not replaced. She was left with a decompression, a small hole in her forehead, just behind the hairline. She continued to have migraines after the operation and, whenever she had an attack, her pulsating brain could be seen to bulge outwards, the decompression becoming more and more tense. At the height of her attack, it stopped pulsating. After she had vomited and slept, the tense brain would return to its normal state.

During attacks sufferers lie still because they know that head movements increase the pain, as do coughing, sneezing, straining and vomiting. The pain of a migraine may be lessened by lying still and being quiet. Some people use ice on the site of pain, others find that a hot-water bottle or pressing the head gives a little relief. This does not mean that the pain is superficial – for instance with stomach-ache we press on the abdominal wall or apply a hot-water bottle, even though the pain arises more deeply.

Not all migraines are accompanied by severe pain and some people manage to work through an attack with the help of pain relievers (see pages 62 and 117).

Loss of appetite, nausea and vomiting
Most people lose their appetite during a migraine attack. This may develop into a dislike of food with a feeling of nausea, leading eventually to vomiting. The smell of food and,

occasionally, even the thought of food, may increase the nausea. Often, vomiting continues until the stomach is empty, and bile or a clear liquid is brought up. Retching is often painful and always unpleasant. Prolonged sickness can lead to dehydration.

Sometimes vomiting heralds the end of an attack; certain people find that a few minutes after they have vomited they begin to feel better.

Children seem more prone to vomiting than adults, with patterns frequently changing over a lifetime. Adults for whom vomiting is not a problem may recall that in childhood their migraines were commonly associated with vomiting. In contrast, however, their adult headaches have become more intense.

Photophobia

A dislike of light (photophobia) is common. The momentary unpleasantness experienced on passing from a darkened room or cinema into the bright sunshine gives an idea of what photophobia feels like. There may be difficulty in focusing and bright objects appear to shimmer, as if in a heat haze. Concentration is also impaired, hence reading becomes impossible.

The degree of photophobia varies. Some people need to take refuge in a totally darkened room, others manage to continue working by taking pain-relieving tablets or wearing dark glasses.

Other symptoms

As well as being very sensitive to light during an attack of migraine, sufferers may become more sensitive to noise and smells (phonophobia and osmophobia). Some people find that during an attack their hearing becomes unpleasantly acute (*hyperacusis*), for example, they can hear the ticking of a clock from another room. Sufferers may become so sensitive to noise that they cannot bear the sound of footsteps coming into their bedroom. Even quiet speech may irritate.

Smells that are usually pleasant, such as coffee, perfume or flowers, may become repugnant. Fried foods, particularly fried onion, are the worst offenders. Cigarette and cigar smoke, lacquers and hairsprays can also cause problems.

During an attack the sufferer's mood may be profoundly lowered. Individuals may become irritable and want to be left alone. This is unusual, because when most people are ill they like the comforting presence of someone nearby. This is yet another symptom suggesting that during a migraine attack the nervous system is irritable and hypersensitive.

Mental processes are slowed: patients often have difficulty in thinking clearly. At a migraine clinic, the nursing sister taking the patients' details reported that during an attack many couldn't remember their home telephone number or the name of their employer.

During an attack people look pale and unwell. Their skin is lax; it may be damp, sweaty or even emit a peculiar odour. There are bags under the eyes. Hands and feet feel cold and sufferers will try to warm themselves because they know that once they are warm, an attack is coming to an end. The bowels are often affected: some people may pass more wind or open their bowels more frequently during an attack, passing loose or even watery stools. Others may become constipated: for them the desire to open their bowels heralds the end of an attack.

Resolution of a migraine attack

About 50 per cent of people with a migraine attack manage to sleep it off. This could be a normal night's sleep, and it may be particularly deep or refreshing. A refreshing sleep need not necessarily be at night. A significant number of people can switch off their attacks by sleeping during the day, with the time taken to do this varying from 30 minutes to six hours, with two and a half hours about average. Typical is one woman who said: 'I pack the kids off to school, tuck myself into bed for three hours, and wake up feeling fine.' Another person said that he usually lunched at home but, if he had a migraine, he would take a siesta for three-quarters of an hour and return to work with a clear head. One doctor dealt with his migraine by sitting and snoozing for 10 to 15 minutes in a quiet dark place (usually the doctors' toilet), which would reduce his headaches sufficiently for him to complete his day's work and go home to bed early.

Observations made at the City of London Migraine Clinic suggest that sleeping, rather than snoozing or dozing, is a more efficient way of ending attacks.

As mentioned before, vomiting may end an attack. This seems more common in children. Many mothers are amazed to discover that 15 minutes after vomiting, their child seems to be back to normal, even wanting to eat again.

Most migraines fade away slowly: the headaches gradually getting less severe over several hours until sufferers realise they have gone. The common pattern is that the patient has an attack during the day, goes to bed early, sleeps, then wakes the following morning with a slight headache, which then gradually disappears.

Migraine postdromes or 'hangovers'

People often mention feeling 'washed out' after a migraine attack. In one study, 50 migraine sufferers were asked about their symptoms after an attack and 47 mentioned variations of mood, muscular weakness, abnormal appetite, tiredness and yawning. Of the 47, 31 had several symptoms that lasted from one hour to four days, the average being for the remainder of the day on which they had the migraine.

Eight of the fifty felt 'high'. In some cases it was a sense of relief; yet in others it was a positive feeling, similar to that in the run up to a migraine, of being able to achieve more than normal. (Some artists and writers value these particular days to do their most creative work.)

More often, however, there was a reported lowering of intellectual capacity, concentration or alertness. Migraine sufferers, in general, use words like 'dopey', 'irritable', 'lifeless', 'unproductive', 'muddled', 'inattentive', 'sluggish', 'not fully alert' or 'distant' to describe how they feel. Routine work is possible, but intellectually demanding tasks are difficult or are avoided together.

Physical tiredness and aching muscles are also common. Some people yawn excessively. One housewife interviewed in the study said that she was capable of preparing meals but could not do much housework. A bank clerk could manage to work during the day but not to play football or squash in the evening. Those whose appetites had been affected found that they could only eat light meals the following day. A few noticed that they passed more urine than normal.

CHAPTER 8

MIGRAINE TYPES

AS STATED in the last chapter, not all attacks of migraine run the same course of five relatively distinct stages of premonitory symptoms, aura, headache, resolution and hangover. In some people one or other stage may predominate or have additional features, which sets their migraine apart from the more frequently encountered forms.

In an attempt to sort out this confusion the International Headache Society has worked out the following system of classification for migraines.★

Migraine without aura (previously known as 'common migraine')

This is characterised by recurring headaches, with attacks lasting from four to 72 hours (or from two to 48 hours in children). The headache is confined to one side of the head in about two-thirds of cases. The headaches, which are of moderate to severe intensity, have a pulsating quality. They are made worse by ordinary physical activity and are associated with nausea, photophobia (exaggerated sensitivity to light) and phonophobia (exaggerated sensitivity to sound). It is, as the name suggests, the most common form of migraine.

Migraines with or without aura may occur almost exclusively

★ The classification system devised by the International Headache Society takes all headaches, not just migraines, into account. It is set out in the headache journal *Cephalalgia* 1988; 8 (suppl 7), pp 1-96.

at a particular time of the menstrual cycle, in which case they are called menstrual migraines.

Migraine with aura (previously known as 'classical migraine')

This is a recurring disorder characterised by attacks of neurological symptoms (the aura) developing gradually over five to 20 minutes and lasting less than an hour. Headache, nausea and photophobia tend to follow these symptoms directly, or after a free interval of less than a hour. The headache usually lasts from four to 72 hours, but may be completely absent.

Auras may be of the following types:
- visual disturbances (see page 79)
- pins and needles and numbness, restricted to one side of the body
- weakness on one side of the body
- difficulties with speech.

There are several other, much rarer, varieties of migraine with aura, as described below.

Migraine with prolonged aura

One or more aura symptoms lasting more than an hour and less than a week. (The diagnosis is made only if results of the special neurological tests are normal.) Most people with this form of migraine have it only occasionally, intermingled with much more frequent attacks with typical aura.

Basilar migraine

See page 81 for aura symptoms.

Migraine aura without headache

It is common in people suffering from migraine with aura that the headache is occasionally absent. This seems to happen more often as people get older: some may find that their headaches disappear completely while their auras continue at (irregular) intervals.

Ophthalmoplegic migraine

In this form, repeated headaches are associated with paralysis of one or more muscles of the eye, giving rise to double vision (*diplopia*).

Retinal migraine

In this form there are repeated attacks of a blind spot or complete blindness in one eye, lasting less than an hour and associated with headache. The defect should disappear completely. The diagnosis of retinal migraine would be made only after specialist assessment.

Cluster headaches

This is a rare type of migraine which differs in many respects from common migraine. It is described in more detail in chapter 13.

Complications of migraine

Status migrainosus

This is an attack of migraine with headache which lasts more than 72 hours despite treatment. It is very rare.

Migrainous infarction

In this form of migraine, the sufferer experiences one or more aura symptoms which are not fully reversible within seven days. It is associated with infarction (injury) of the brain tissue. Migrainous infarction is rare but if the symptoms last for longer than usual, medical help should be sought.

CHAPTER 9

WHO GETS MIGRAINES?

IN EVERY community where it has been looked for, migraine sufferers have been found. The actual proportion varies according to how the investigators defined migraine and how thorough they were. A pitfall of the early studies was that calculations were based on how many people consulted their doctors with migraine. This led to an appreciable underestimation: many migraine sufferers *never* consult their doctors about their condition.★

Factors influencing migraine

Age

It used to be thought that migraines began in the teens and ended at the menopause in women, and in the 50s in men. However, it has become apparent that migraines may begin in childhood and persist into the 70s. Migraine is, however, predominantly a younger person's condition: the average age of those attending one migraine clinic was 38. Most sufferers have their first attack of migraine before they are 20, with perhaps one in eight having their first symptoms before the age of ten. A first attack of migraine after 50 is unusual but not unknown.

★ An average estimate of the proportion of the population who suffers from migraine without aura ('common migraine') is one in 10, with about one in 100 being affected by migraine with aura ('classical' migraine).

Migraine in childhood

At least 3 to 4 per cent of children suffer from migraines. One study found that one in three children with migraines developed their first symptoms before the age of five; even babies have been described as having attacks. The City of London Migraine Clinic was surprised to find that one in ten of its new patients were aged 16 or under.

Despite the widely held belief that children cannot describe their symptoms clearly, a child aged five with a migraine, if allowed to speak, can often give a vivid description of an attack.

As in adults, migraines may occur with or without a visual warning. Childhood migraine differs from the adult form in its association with attacks of abdominal pain: three in four children with a migraine experience these, which are centred on the navel. In some children, the abdominal pain may be the dominant or only symptom. However, it is still disputed whether recurrent abdominal pains in childhood are migrainous in origin. Some certainly are not. Children's migraine attacks are often shorter and may end quickly, often after vomiting.

The same factors that trigger migraine in adults can trigger attacks in children, and children will respond to the same treatment. Weighing less, however, they need smaller doses of drugs and should not be given aspirin (see page 63). During the course of childhood attacks, migraines usually become less severe: after ten years of migraines one-third to one-half of sufferers report that their headaches have either gone completely or have become much reduced.

Schoolteachers should know about a child's migraines, especially if treatment involves taking tablets. If the child is allowed to rest in a quiet, dark room from the beginning of an attack this may help to end the attacks more quickly.

Migraine in the elderly

Migraine may not disappear at 50 years of age, as was once thought: 8 per cent of new patients at the City of London Migraine Clinic are over 60. Migraines can stop at virtually any age or change their pattern. Sufferers may lose their headaches but retain their nausea, or have fewer stomach symptoms but retain their headaches. Others lose their headaches but retain their visual warnings. How and why patterns change is not known.

Gender

Women are two to three times more likely to suffer from migraines than men, with women in their reproductive years the most affected. Menstruation and the oral contraceptive pill make migraines more likely. The effect of hormone replacement therapy (HRT) still needs to be evaluated.

Pregnancy

Mysteriously, migraines usually improve during pregnancy: two-thirds of migraine sufferers are completely free of attacks during the last six months of pregnancy.

Menopause

In the past it was thought that migraine was worse during 'the change'. However, a study in Oxford showed that migraines at this time of life could be better, worse, or even the same as before. The menopause may be associated with depression, anxiety or hot flushes, all making migraines more difficult to cope with.

Hormonal factors are not responsible for all women's migraine: in some they play no part, in others they play a major role, but in most they are a contributory factor.

Heredity

Migraine sufferers have about a 60 per cent chance of having a relative with migraine; people without migraine have only a 10 per cent chance of having an affected relative. From these figures there seems little doubt that migraines run in families, and some researchers have chosen to interpret this as proof that migraines are inherited genetically.

Results from the few studies done in twins give only tentative evidence to support this. Some attacks occurring in families, however, may result from younger family members adopting from their elders' ways of responding to stress, but there is no scientific support for such a belief.

A migraine personality?

The idea of a personality type which is more prone to migraines has a long history, and a whole lexicon exists to describe the 'typical' migraine sufferer: intelligent, hardworking, upright, over-conscientious, rigid, ambitious and perfectionist.

Most of these are considered virtues – could it be that people who suffer from migraines are somehow special? The problem is that many in the medical profession who write about migraines have a particular interest in the condition because they are themselves sufferers. Thus, the picture they paint of 'the migraine personality' may have more to do with how they see themselves and their patients than with the generality of migraine sufferers. Against this exclusive view of migraines are the findings from community studies where attempts have been made to assess everyone, not just those who consult their doctor. These have not confirmed the existence of 'a migraine personality'. Migraine does not seem to be associated with either higher intelligence or higher social class though distorted figures may appear to reveal this. It is true, however, that in many societies, higher social groups are more likely to be able to afford or seek medical treatment and are also more likely to be able to articulate their symptoms to a doctor, all of which contributes to erroneous figures about the true pattern of migraine.

Famous migraine sufferers

It should not surprise us if some great names from the past suffered from migraines. If one in ten of the population are prone to attacks then so too should have been one in ten artists, writers, statesmen and so on. Those who suffered from migraines included Julius Caesar, Peter the Great, Mary Tudor, Edward Gibbon, John Calvin, Immanuel Kant, Friedrich Nietzsche, Blaise Pascal, Linnaeus, Sir John Herschel, Thomas Jefferson, Ulysses Grant, George Eliot and Sigmund Freud.

The neurologist E M R Critchley has claimed that the following have all used their own experience of migraines in their writings: William Shakespeare, John Dryden, Miguel de Cervantes, Alexander Pope, Jonathan Swift, Lewis Carroll, Anthony Trollope, G K Chesterton, Rudyard Kipling, Ralph Waldo Emerson, W S Gilbert, Mary Stewart, Pamela Hansford Johnson, and Arthur Ransome.

LEWIS CARROLL

'Do I look very pale?' said Tweedledum, coming up to have his helmet tied on. (He *called* it a helmet, though it certainly looked much more like a saucepan.) 'Well – yes – a *little,*' Alice replied gently. 'I'm very brave, generally,' he went on in a low voice, only to-day I happen to have a headache.'

From: *Through the Looking Glass*

Lewis Carroll suffered from migraines, and symptoms of migraine may be spotted in both *Alice's Adventures in Wonderland* and *Through the Looking Glass.* Alice's disconcerting changes in size are similar to the disturbances of vision occasionally experienced by people during a migraine aura. The slow disappearance of the Cheshire Cat, beginning with the end of its tail, 'and ending with the grin, which remained some time after the rest of it had gone', is reminiscent of the patchy loss of vision that occurs during a migrating aura.

Migraines in history

The stresses of Western civilisation are blamed for many of the problems that befall modern man, but for once they cannot be wholly blamed for migraine. Migraine seems to have been around for as long as records have been kept. The British Museum has a papyrus with hieroglyphics denoting a one-sided headache.

Aretaeus was a physician, born c.AD80 in Cappodocia (now Asiatic Turkey), who lived and practised medicine, first in Alexandria, then in Rome. He based his practice on Hippocratic principles, dividing disease into acute and chronic elements. He distinguished cephalalgia, a headache lasting days, from cephalea, a headache persisting for longer. He is also credited with giving the first good description of migraine, which he called heterocrania – a pain affecting either the right or left side of the head or both together. One hundred years later (in the second century AD), the famous physician Galen coined the term 'hemicrania'. The word 'migraine' is a corruption of hemicrania, which is why some people maintain that the condition should be pronounced mee-grain. The word 'migraine' first appeared in French; the early English equivalent was 'megrim'.

Migraines during work

Figures from the Department of Health and Social Security in England in the mid-1980s showed that nearly 500,000 working days were lost each year because of migraine. Although the figure seems high it is almost certainly an underestimate as most migraines do not last long enough to warrant a medical certificate.

A study conducted in a food factory employing 2,000 people in the south of England revealed the incidence of migraine was 6 per cent and, over eight months, 281 working days were lost. Some 98 patients reported a total of 111 attacks during these eight months; 36 occurred at work and 75 outside working hours.

We do not know what the effects on performance and productivity are: many sufferers complete their day's work in spite of pain and then go home and sleep their attacks off. It is possible that migraines make them less efficient.

CHAPTER 10

THEORIES

THE CAUSE of migraine remains a mystery, but with increasingly sophisticated tests becoming available more is now known about what happens in the brain during a migraine attack. This is not the same as knowing the cause, but it is a good beginning.

Blood flow studies

Migraine with an aura

Studies suggest that during the aura there is a reduction in the amount of blood flowing to the brain. This decrease starts at the back of the brain progressing forward at a speed of about 2 to 3 mm a minute.

A minimum level of blood supply is needed for the brain to function properly, and if it goes below a certain level, symptoms occur. The occipital lobes of the brain which are responsible for vision are where the problems begin: the most frequent auras entail visual disturbance. Too little blood further forward in the brain accounts for the symptoms of numbness, pins and needles and weakness that affect the face, arms and legs.

The reduction in blood flow may precede the aura by minutes and flow may still be reduced after the aura has gone and the typical headache begun. Usually, however, the headache is associated with a rebound increase in blood flow to higher than normal levels. Again the correlation between blood flow and symptoms may not be exact: the period of increased blood flow may last longer than the headache.

Migraine without an aura

Blood flow studies have been far more equivocal in people having common migraines. The pattern may be either that a headache follows an increased blood flow to the brain; or that headaches are not associated with any change in blood flow at all.

These contradictory findings result from investigations in Scandinavia and the USA, the former claiming a reduction and the latter an increased blood flow.

Vascular v. neurological theory

Specialists have been arguing for the last hundred years whether the primary problem stems from the blood vessels or the brain itself. The 'vascular' theory holds that the blood vessels supplying the brain shut down for their own reasons and that the brain's reduced functions are affected as a result of the decrease in blood supply. (This is analogous to blood vessels in the hands closing down when exposed to the cold – without ill effects.)

In the 'neurological' theory migraine is supposed to begin in the brain tissue itself, and the blood vessels shut down as a secondary response to the changes in the brain. The proponents of the neurological theory say it is analogous to someone going pale with fear – the emotion arises first in the central nervous system and then blood vessels constrict. (Similarly, blood vessels may dilate with emotion, as in blushing. In both these cases the effects on the vessels are secondary.)

Neurotransmitters

For whatever reason the blood flow to the brain decreases during an attack of migraine, neurotransmitters are bound to be directly involved. These chemical messengers of the brain create changes in the functions of the brain and in the blood vessels that supply it. Could abnormalities in the levels of neurotransmitters be the cause of migraine? Certainly many of the drugs that are effective in preventing migraine are known to block the actions of neurotransmitters. The group of neurotransmitters most intensively studied have been the amines: serotonin (5-hydroxytryptamine – 5HT for short), the catecholamines (noradrenaline, adrenaline, and dopamine), histamine, tyramine and phenylethylamine (see page 135).

Platelets

These tiny cells that circulate in the blood stream are responsible for plugging breaches in the lining of blood vessels. During a migraine attack they release the chemical serotonin (5HT), which has a powerful constricting effect on blood vessels and also acts as a neurotransmitter between brain cells (see above). One school of thought places the primary cause of migraine down to platelets.

Allergy

Studies done on children with migraine attacks have suggested that some attacks may be due to food allergy. Similarly, one study described adults with migraines who were resistant to the usual treatment but improved when given drugs known to reduce the body's allergic response. Confirmation of these findings is still awaited, although research was carried out more than five years ago.

PART 4

MANAGING MIGRAINES

CHAPTER 11

MANAGING MIGRAINES: ON YOUR OWN

THE CAUSE of migraines is unknown and so far no cure has been found. This may seem a disheartening way to begin a chapter on managing migraines, yet steps can be taken to lessen the severity of a migraine attack once it has begun. Recognising what triggers an attack may allow you to avoid them completely.

The acute attack

- Stop what you are doing and retire to a quiet, darkened room. Some people try 'working through' an attack: a few manage it, but many more are unsuccessful.
- Try to go to sleep. Studies have shown that those who manage to sleep recover better than those who only rest or doze (see page 85).
- Keep warm with the help of blankets, hot-water bottle or a heater. Some sufferers find that a hot bath helps.
- Try pressing on the site of the pain or holding a hot-water bottle or ice-pack there which can reduce the pain.
- Take simple analgesics: either aspirin 600-900mg (two or three tablets) or paracetamol 1000mg (two tablets) *early in the attack* and repeat at 4- to 6-hourly intervals if necessary. (See page 120 for more details about taking these and other forms of medication during an attack.)

Avoiding triggers

'Many patients consider their migraines to occur spontaneously and without cause. Such a view leads, scientifically to absurdity, emotionally to fatalism, and therapeutically to impotence. We must assume that all attacks of migraine have real and discoverable determinants, however difficult their elucidation may be.'

From: *Migraine: Understanding the Common Disorder* by Oliver Sachs, Pan, 1985, London.

There are two things you should bear in mind as you read this chapter. First, triggers do not consistently provoke attacks, just as it doesn't always rain when there are clouds in the sky. Secondly, two or three triggers may act together.

It may be useful to separate the internal factors that predispose people to develop attacks from the triggers that set off individual attacks. These internal factors may vary with time; for example, some women find that drinking red wine in the week before their period regularly induces an attack, whereas drinking red wine during the rest of the cycle is perfectly safe. Other people find that having recently had an attack of migraine protects them for a certain time – even if they are exposed to their usual triggers. It is as if there were an internal level, a kind of thermostat, that determines whether the triggers acting at a particular time will induce an attack.

If you started this book at the beginning, you will realise that the factors that cause migraines are the same as those that cause 'Everyday Headaches' (chapter 1). This is an important and relatively recent concept: the factors responsible for ordinary headaches may induce migraine attacks in those who are susceptible to them. These triggers will now be described in greater detail. A checklist appears on page 112.

Food: too little or too late

Many people know that they are liable to have an attack of migraine if they go without food or eat only a snack instead of a full meal. Delaying a meal by an hour or so can have the same effect, as can dieting.

CASE HISTORY

A bachelor found that his migraines disappeared once he was married. When single he used to have irregular meals and often went out 'drinking with the boys'. After marriage he ate regular meals at home, drank less and put on weight – a combination that drastically reduced his migraine attacks.

A slice of toast for breakfast will keep you going for only about an hour and lunch may well be five or six hours away. Some people eat a sandwich for lunch without getting up from their desks. Try taking some time away from your work, even if it is

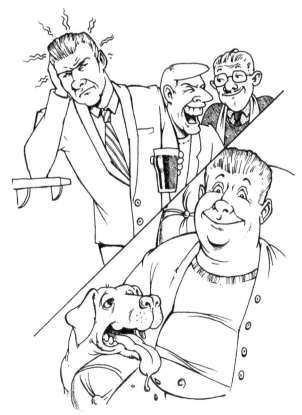

[Figure 8: A 'before and after' view of the benefits of married life.]

only a few minutes, to relax a little and perhaps eat something more substantial. Missing lunch to save 20 to 30 minutes one day may be a false economy if migraine puts you out of action the next.

Thin people may be more prone to hunger-related migraine: those with a 'lean and hungry look' should eat more frequently. If people need to diet they should eat a little less at each meal, aiming to lose only half an ounce a day, or nearly a pound a month – which is about the rate at which people gain weight. Drastic dieting to lose weight can increase the severity and frequency of migraine attacks.

Dietary factors

Many foodstuffs and beverages have been identified as causing migraines. The more frequently cited include:

- chocolate
- alcohol (with red wine and port the worst offenders)
- cheese (especially ripe cheeses: cottage cheese and other light cheeses rarely cause problems)
- citrus fruits
- nuts
- meats, including sausages
- dairy products
- coffee and tea
- foods containing monosodium glutamate.

It may be that cheese delays stomach emptying so that nourishment does not get into the system and the ultimate effect is the same as eating too little food.

Chocolate may be taken as a substitute for food and not provide sufficient calories. Another explanation for chocolate's effect is that a craving for sweet foods may be one of the premonitory symptoms (see page 78) and to satisfy this craving chocolate is eaten. So the migraine attack may have already started, but chocolate, an 'innocent bystander', gets the blame.

Even if someone is prone to alcohol-induced migraine, not all alcoholic drinks will have the same effect; for example, red wine may be worse than white, and beer and sherry worse than whisky. It is important to find out which type of alcohol, if any, agrees with you. Many people avoid alcohol alogether. If you worry about being too conspicuous you can drink bitter lemon, soda, ginger ale, or an alcohol-free wine or beer. Some people find they can drink alcohol without causing a migraine if they eat a little food first.

If you think that anything in your diet is causing your attacks of migraine then try omitting it for a month. If this makes no difference then re-introduce it and omit another dietary suspect.

Sleep: too little or too much

For many people, a bad night's sleep or its opposite – a lie-in at the weekend – can result in an attack of migraine. A lie-in does not even have to be very long. An extra hour or two can be sufficient to provoke a headache or a migraine. It is a mystery why too much sleep causes migraines, although it is interesting that alcohol, which increases the depth and duration of sleep, may also cause migraine. Many years ago 'sleep rationing' was tried as a treatment for migraine, with some success.

Those for whom sleep may be a factor can experiment, allowing themselves perhaps an extra hour of sleep on Saturdays and Sundays. If they remain migraine-free for several weekends, they can extend their sleep by an hour and a half, and then two hours, to determine how much extra they can tolerate before an attack is provoked.

Going to bed late on one night or on two or three consecutive nights can also provoke migraine attacks.

Female hormones

Women know that attacks are more likely to occur in the week before their periods when they experience other premenstrual symptoms, such as feeling irritable and tense. Some women retain fluids: their abdomens and breasts swell and their clothes feel tighter. This is the time to be particularly careful about avoiding triggers – for example, missed meals and alcohol.

The oral contraceptive pill can increase the frequency and severity of attacks in women who already suffer from migraines. Some women on intermittent treatment – three weeks on the pill and one week off – may have attacks only during the week when they are off the pill. They may be helped by taking the pill continuously. Migraines may get worse when hormones are given for the menopausal or post-menopausal symptoms. In these cases a doctor looking after a patient with a migraine may have to work in conjunction with her gynaecologist. For some women it may be necessary to stop hormonal treatment altogether.

WARNING

If a woman has a change in the pattern of her migraines while taking the pill, then she should consult her doctor urgently. It may be a warning of an impending stroke, in which case she should stop taking the pill immediately.

Local pains in the head and neck

Pain in the eyes or difficulties with focusing, pain arising from the sinuses, the teeth, or even the upper part of the neck, particularly in the middle-aged and elderly, may trigger migraine attacks. In these cases the appropriate measures, for example, physiotherapy for a painful neck, can reduce migraine attacks. Dentists can help by reducing local pains (usually related to the jaw), impacted wisdom teeth, or an abnormal 'bite'.

Environmental factors

Excessive noise, heat, light, and odours, pleasant or otherwise, can provoke a migraine attack. Odours include cigarette and cigar smoke, paints, hairsprays, perfumes, soaps and occasionally specific flowers. Certain types of weather may also induce attacks.

One activity may combine several noxious environmental stimuli. Shopping, when the stores are hot, where there is fluorescent lighting and it is moderately stressful, is a good example. Going to the cinema may induce migraines.

Some triggers, such as the weather, cannot be changed, but if heat is a problem, for instance at parties, then evasive action is possible. You could stand near a window perhaps, and leave early. Often centrally-heated rooms can be humidified by having a bowl of water or a plant in the room. In a hotel bedroom, a damp towel or a little water in the wash basin will have the same effect. Dark glasses reduce the intensity of bright lights. Ear plugs may help to reduce noise, especially on an enforced noisy journey.

Exercise and travel

Hard physical exercise can trigger migraines in some people. Try taking glucose tablets before and immediately after exertion and then eating a sandwich when the exercise is over.

Travel is another activity combining several possible migraine triggers. Often going away on holiday is accompanied by excitement, but there are steps you can take to avoid an attack.

- To avoid being under pressure allow yourself an extra half-hour to get ready.
- Do not skip meals. Have something to eat before leaving home and again when you arrive at the airport, railway station, bus terminal or wherever.
- If you suffer from travel sickness take the appropriate tablets and have a light meal half an hour before setting out. This is particularly important on an aeroplane journey, where the meals are often delayed and the lower oxygen pressure can further contribute to a headache. Travel sickness may provoke an attack of migraine in both adults and children. Even if you don't usually suffer from travel sickness the tablets can help prevent an attack of migraine if subsequent meals are delayed or unappetising.
- Avoid alcohol if it provokes attacks.

Allergy

Theories linking migraine with allergy were very popular earlier this century and have made something of a comeback recently. Medical opinion is currently divided over whether allergy is an important cause of migraine.

If you think you may be allergic to a certain food or group of foods, then follow the directions given earlier in this chapter under 'Dietary factors' (page 108).

Psychological factors

Many sufferers recognise that their attacks follow a period of stress, frustration or annoyance. Interestingly, migraines strike *after* and not *during* a period of stress: the business executive develops his or her migraine on Saturday or Sunday; the vicar on Monday.

Coping with stress

Talking with someone who is not part of your immediate circle can make you feel less stressed and so reduce your migraines. Many problems stem from work. If you are expected to do two people's work or to produce 'tomorrow's work yesterday', then it is time for a talk with your boss.

Consider ways of relaxing, but select one that suits you. Many people find jogging, swimming or golf helpful; others relax by reading a book or by watching television. There are a number of 'schools' of relaxation, one or more of which may suit you.

Details of progressive relaxation are given on page 60. Details of other treatments that may reduce stress are included in the appendix dealing with complementary therapies. Relaxation should not be limited to a few minutes a day but should extend throughout the working day and ideally extend to your whole life.

A checklist of precipitating factors for migraine headaches

Have a careful look at this list of possible triggers for your migraine headaches, but note that they may not invariably provoke attacks.

1. *Lack of food:*
   Fasting
   Delaying or missing meals
   Too little food (for example, a snack or salad)

2. *Specific foods:*
   Chocolate
   Alcohol (red wine and port are the worst offenders)
   Cheese (especially ripe cheeses: cottage cheese and other light cheeses rarely cause problems)
   Citrus fruits
   Nuts
   Meats, including sausages
   Dairy products
   Coffee and tea
   Foods containing monosodium glutamate

3. *Sleep:*
   Too much
   Too little

4. *Hormones (women only):*
   During or before period
   Menopausal symptoms
   The pill

5. *Local pains in head or neck:*
   Eyes
   Sinuses
   Neck
   Teeth or jaw

6. **Environmental factors:**
   Heat
   Cold
   Light
   Noise
   Cinema
   Shopping
   Parties
   Odours

7. **Exercise or travel**

8. **Allergy**

9. **Stress**

A practical approach

If you can't identify a trigger from this list, keep a record of attacks, paying attention to the preceding 12 to 24 hours. The items you should list in your headache diary are given on page 58.

A regular pattern of attacks may suggest precipitating factors. When do your attacks start? If you wake with a migraine then dietary factors the evening before, sleep disturbances or neck problems (especially in the middle-aged) should be considered. If attacks begin during the morning you should pay attention to insufficient food at breakfast, tension due to travelling, or conditions at work. Attacks coming on later in the day may also be due to the work environment (which could be physical or psychological) or an inadequate lunch.

Finding a consistent pattern does not always lead directly to the trigger. For example, migraines occurring regularly at the weekend may be caused by a late Friday evening meal, undue pressure at work during the last two weekdays, alcohol on Friday or Saturday night, or sleeping longer or more deeply at the weekend when you are relaxed.

If you cannot identify a single trigger for your attacks, then think of combinations. Some people can drink red wine without problems unless they're tired – when alcohol provokes their migraines. Parties may provoke a migraine. In the rush to get there an afternoon snack may be missed and the food on offer may be unsuitable or insufficient. Then there may be added factors, such as heat, noise and alcohol.

Obviously if you can identify one or more triggers, you should try to avoid them, although this may not always be possible.

CHAPTER 12

MANAGING MIGRAINES: DRUGS AND DOCTORS

TODAY, unfortunately, drugs have mostly bad connotations: people are afraid of becoming addicted to what their doctors prescribe them. Most medication can have unpleasant, occasionally even harmful side-effects, but taken under supervision and sensibly, the risk is small. The right medication, taken at the right time, can be highly beneficial. See also chapter 6 for details on medication for headaches and the appendix for the complementary approaches to treating migraine.

A few tips

- Keep to the dosage prescribed. Some people take one instead of two tablets, or four instead of two. Applying this rule to spectacles you will appreciate that half-strength or double-strength glasses are not necessarily helpful. Having taken the number of tablets advised, note carefully any response, when it started, and how long it lasted. Also note any side-effects.
- When you next see your doctor you can then report accurately, benefit or otherwise, on the effects of his or her prescription.
- Not all colours suit everyone, and the same is true for medication. For those who find that some tablets are too large and stick in their throats, there may be capsules or lozenge-shaped tablets, which can be swallowed more easily. Effervescent preparations suit some people while others find the gas nauseating. Your doctor should be able to advise you about different forms of the same drug.

- Tablets should *always* be taken with a drink so that they go down quickly and completely. This should also make unpleasant-tasting tablets less so.
- Tablets taken before a meal are more quickly absorbed than those taken afterwards. A fatty meal slows down absorption even more. When it is important to get a drug into your system quickly, which is the case with a migraine, tablets should be taken on an empty stomach. Swill the tablets down with water or a warm drink (which dissolves the tablets more easily and is soothing) and sit quietly for about half an hour until the tablets are absorbed. Then have something to eat. In this way you may be able to reduce or even eliminate the head pain and the nausea.
- Take the tablets at the first sign of a migraine. If you wait until the migraine has built up, there is very little that can be done other than going to bed and sleeping it off. Disturbances of vision are the commonest warning symptoms of an impending attack; others are listed on page 76. If you don't get any clear-cut warnings (and only about 10 to 15 per cent of people do) take effective treatment as soon as possible after your headache starts.

  Many people are reluctant to take tablets early, believing that the attack will not get any worse or will go away by itself. The necessity for early medication, however, is that as an attack progresses intestinal movement become slower, and the pylorus, the outlet from the stomach, may close. This delays or even prevents the absorption of drugs taken by mouth. Another reason for taking tablets early is that analgesics have only a certain effect; let us say that they can treat pain up to a level 'X'. If the pain has risen to levels of 2X or 3X, then the tablets will not work.

The principles of treatment

An important discovery made at the City of London Migraine Clinic was that by taking the anti-nausea drug metoclopramide, followed by pain-relieving tablets (two paracetamol or three aspirin), many attacks were aborted, even when well established. Metoclopramide has the added advantage of promoting gastric emptying and normal peristalsis. (Nausea can be stopped by using suppositories, and the analgesics then taken by mouth.)

During one year 280 patients were treated with this combination at the migraine clinic. Nine out of ten of them were either symptom-free or had only slight, residual headaches after an average of three and a quarter hours. Another useful observation was made: the patients who slept recovered better than those who only snoozed or dozed.

When this discovery was applied to a food factory, 35 out of 36 workers with migraine were back at the bench within an hour. Why was their recovery so much quicker than at the migraine clinic? One possible explanation was that they had earlier treatment at the factory, having only to walk to the nursing station. In the centre of London a worker has to decide, perhaps reluctantly, to leave the office and then to travel to the clinic, therefore the treatment would be given much later in the attack. If this is so then it supports the advice that treatment should be given early. It also suggests that after taking the tablets the person should wait for some effect (about half an hour) before returning to work.

A DISCOVERY IN NEW YORK

Dr David Coddon, working at Mount Sinai Hospital in New York, was impressed by the effects of sleep on migraines. When called to a young patient who was having a migraine attack he decided to give him an injection (he was too ill to take tablets). He decided on chlorpromazine to counteract the pallor and vomiting and a hypnotic, amylobarbitone sodium, for the pain. The boy fell into a deep sleep for about two hours. It worked like magic!

He has now treated many hundreds of patients by giving them an intravenous injection of a combination of promazine and two barbiturates: a quick- and a slow-acting one. In his experience if the patient sleeps for three or four hours after the injection, he or she will wake feeling very much better. Here the treatment is directed against the main symptoms of migraines: nausea, pain and the need to sleep. Injections are the last resort, used only if patients cannot take tablets by mouth. (Suppositories may also be used.)

Drugs used during an attack

For the headache

Aspirin and paracetamol (See also pages 62-3)
Take a careful look at the label on the bottle or packet of your usual headache tablets: more often than not you will read aspirin or paracetamol or both. Singly or in combination these two drugs are excellent for mild and moderate pains, regardless of where they arise. Other drugs may be added, for example, codeine (which increases the pain-relieving effect of aspirin), a sedative, an antihistamine, or something to soothe the stomach.

Most adults need between 600 and 900mg of aspirin (two or three tablets). Paracetamol comes in 500mg tablets: most adults need 1000mg, or two tablets.

If the attack has not gone within four hours – about how long these tablets last – you should take a second dose, the same as the first. If that fails do not take any more tablets during that attack. Children should not be given aspirin and the dose of paracetamol should be scaled down according to weight.

For the nausea

Antihistamine
Antihistamine tablets, commonly used for travel sickness, can stop or reduce the nausea that is a common symptom of migraines. If nausea makes taking tablets by mouth impossible, then suppositories containing similar drugs are available. Once the nausea settles down, pain-relieving tablets may be taken by mouth.

Metoclopramide
During a migraine the movements of the stomach and the intestines slow down, delaying the absorption of food, drink,

and, most importantly during an attack, drugs. (The upper part of the small intestine is where most substances are absorbed through the gut wall to reach the blood stream, by which chemicals reach the brain.) Nausea is more likely to increase to vomiting if the stomach is full of undigested food. Metoclopramide increases the movement of the intestines and also has an effect on the brain which reduces nausea. It should not be taken by children.

Domperidone
Domperidone acts similarly to metoclopramide by emptying the stomach and increasing the activity of the muscles of the gut.

Prochlorperazine
Prochlorperazine, like metoclopramide, reduces nausea and can be given rectally.

Other drugs

Ergotamine
For some, the ergot family of drugs is most effective in aborting migraine attacks. Over the years its reputation has suffered because of its side-effects, but in healthy individuals with healthy blood vessels and normal blood pressure, these should be rare. Gangrene is an extremely rare complication: though people with this side-effect have usually taken 10, 20 or more times the recommended dose. Doses of 6 to 8mg per attack and 10 to 12mg per week should not be exceeded. Ergotamine treatment should not be repeated at intervals of less than four days.

Ergotamine comes in several different forms: tablets to swallow, tablets to dissolve under the tongue, aerosols that deliver the drug by puff (inhaled through the mouth in the same way that asthma drugs are), injections or suppositories for insertion after the bowels have been opened. Like other drugs used for aborting attacks ergotamine must be taken early.

The common side-effects of ergotamine are nausea, vomiting, cold hands and feet, muscle cramps and abdominal pain – symptoms which wear off after two or three hours.

Too much ergotamine may itself cause headaches, as discovered by Dr Marcia Wilkinson at the City of London Migraine Clinic. If someone takes ergotamine tartrate tablets for a mild headache and repeats the dose six or seven hours later, a headache due to the ergotamine may develop. Ergotamine can also cause a headache the following morning.

Ergot headaches respond to ergot – if another ergotamine is taken to counteract the headache, then the sufferer may get hooked and will need to take at least one tablet a day. Many people with headaches from an overdose of ergotamine tartrate are taking three, four or even more of these tablets a day. Sometimes they need admission to hospital to wean them off the drug. Ergot is not recommended for children.

Drugs between attacks

The frequency and severity of attacks of migraine vary widely – from once or twice a month to once or twice a year. If you are getting more than two severe attacks a month, then prophylactic (or 'interval') treatment may be considered. This should be medically supervised. The drugs below are those used:

beta blockers
   atenolol
   metoprolol
   nadolol
   propranolol
   timolol

serotonin receptor antagonists
   methysergide
   pizotifen

prostaglandin inhibitors (non-steroidal anti-inflammatory
   drugs)
   diclofenac
   naproxen

others
  amitriptyline
  clonidine
  feverfew
  sedatives (occasionally used, but not advisable)

Antidepressants have been found to be of value in people who are depressed, and they have also been found to be effective in migraines even when depression is not a feature.

Feverfew

'Take of feverfew one handful, warm it in a frying-pan, apply it twice or thrice hot; this cures a hemicrania. And the crude herb applied to the top of the head, cures the headache.'

From: *Compleat Herbal of Physical Plants* by Pechey, 1707.

The headache-relieving properties of feverfew have been known for a long time. This eighteenth-century herbal did not suggest eating the leaves of this common weed, but recently, carefully performed medical trials suggest that eating three fresh leaves a day reduces the frequency and intensity of migraine. Nausea and vomiting may also be lessened.

A generalised soreness of the mouth and ulceration may be a problem. Some migraine sufferers claim to avoid these symptoms by eating the leaves in a sandwich. Otherwise no untoward effects have been found in people taking feverfew for long periods of time.

It is important to choose the right feverfew plant: *Tanacetum parthenium*, the wild feverfew plant with the yellow–white head. Tablets containing the same amount of active ingredient, 25mg, can also be bought, if you do not wish to, or cannot, grow the plant. One tablet should be taken daily.

Doctors

Is there any point in seeing your doctor if you have a migraine? If you are coping on your own without problems, then probably not. (You would be in good company: one study found that less than half those who had a migraine consulted a doctor about it at sometime during their lives.)

Some people with severe migraines find that they lose faith in their ability to cope and in the effectiveness of the medication they have been taking. In these circumstances it can be useful to have a second opinion, the doctor's, and to transfer your care, however temporarily, to someone else. Remember that it is you and you alone who has to cope with the condition long-term. Some people say that as soon as they have decided to see a doctor they begin to feel better.

Do not go shopping around looking for migraine cures; at present there are none. What your general practitioner or specialist will be able to do is to help you identify any triggers for your attacks, recommend ways of avoiding them, coping with them when you to get them and ensuring that you benefit from the best treatments available. At present there is a whole range of new drugs being investigated – it could well be that one or more of them will turn out to be useful.

A minimum of ten years elapses between the birth of a new drug and its prescription by doctors. The government has laid down the strictest precautions and prolonged trials to ensure the safety of medical products. Many drugs fail at various stages of their development.

What can you do before going to the doctor?

Keep a record of your attacks and take it with you. Note as many details of the attacks as you can. Also important are the names of any tablets you have tried and whether they worked and any factors which you think might have provoked your attacks. Chapter 6 gives more details about seeking medical advice, and some questions you may be asked.

PART 5

RARE CONDITIONS AND FUTURE RESEARCH

CHAPTER 13

CLUSTER HEADACHES

THIS IS a rare type of headache, which differs in several respects from the more common migraine described in the previous six chapters. The following case report provides the main features.

CASE HISTORY

A 48-year-old civil servant had suffered from recurrent headaches from the age of 33. He thought that his headaches were associated with autumn, although they did not always occur then. Between the spells he was totally symptom-free and enjoyed good health.

During a cluster, his headaches occurred every night for six to eight weeks, usually waking him with remarkable regularity at 2.30am. The pain always felt as if it was coming from the right eye. It would build up slowly over five to ten minutes, after which he would get out of bed and pace the bedroom. If he looked in the bathroom mirror then he could see that the affected eye was red and the eyelids swollen. Sometimes tears would stream from his right eye. His right nostril was blocked.

The pain would become so severe that he did not know what to do with himself. Sometimes he might press on his forehead and eye with his hands; at times he wanted to 'bash his head against the wall', so intense was the pain. After about three-quarters of an hour, the pain would disappear, leaving him shaken, with a dull ache round his eye lasting a few more hours. Attacks occasionally occurred during the day, when they were usually provoked by alcohol. Because of this he rarely 'touched a drop' during spells.

Nothing from his past medical history or family history suggested a cause for his headaches. Before he was correctly diagnosed he had seen several specialists but none of the recommended treatments had helped his pain.

Original descriptions

Although migraine headaches have been known about for 2,400 years, cluster headaches (or migrainous neuralgia) were not recognised until about 1830, when Mauritz Romberg, a German neurologist, gave a hazy description of them. The first full

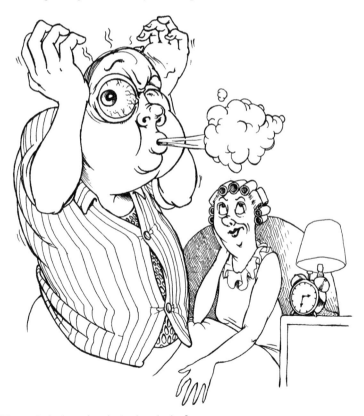

[Figure 9: A view of a cluster headache.]

description was given in 1926 by Wilfred Harris, a London neurologist, who called it 'periodic migrainous neuralgia'. It was also delineated by Dr Bayard Taylor Horton in the United States, where it became known as Horton's cephalgia. Other names proposed for it have included Vidian's neuralgia, Schluder's neuralgia and, as late as 1956, Sir Charles Symonds devoted an article to it entitled 'A Particular Variety of Headache'.

Symonds' article is of special interest because he records how a patient discovered that an injection of ergotamine before going to sleep stopped his attacks. Another eminent neurologist had advised the patient to inject himself at the beginning of an attack, but without any success. The patient tried an experiment using the injection preventively. Thus he contributed to our knowledge of treatment of this condition by discovering that injections had to be given *some hours before an attack was due*.

Incidence and gender

Men comprise the majority of those who suffer with cluster headaches – only one in five is female; most are middle-aged, with the condition usually commencing between the ages of 20 and 40, which is 10 to 15 years later than the onset of migraine. Some people find that their clusters occur only at certain times of the year, although the reason for this is unknown. Alcohol and nitroglycerine (used to treat angina) are known to precipitate attacks.

The attacks typically occur during night-time sleep, sometimes waking the sufferer so regularly that for a while the headaches were called 'alarm clock headaches'. Some sufferers still volunteer, 'It is as if an alarm clock has gone off inside my head'.

During a cluster headache the same eye is always affected. In the case history given above the pain was right-sided, but it can affect either eye. Only very rarely does the headache change from one side to the other, and then only in different cluster periods.

Diagnosis

Because the condition is so rare – perhaps only one in 10,000 people are affected – few doctors have seen enough cases to be able to diagnose the condition confidently. Long delays before the correct diagnosis is made are common.

Origin of pain

Whether the pain comes from local blood vessels dilating, or from the nerves supplying these vessels, is unknown. Tests measuring skin temperature have shown that the region around the affected eye is warmer, but there is a cold area in the forehead above the eye – presumably because of diminished blood supply. Once again, the cause for this is unknown. Most sufferers discover by experience that drinking alcohol can provoke an attack within 20 to 40 minutes when they are in the cluster phase, in contrast to the ordinary migraine headache, where alcohol produces an attack the following morning. The time elapsing between drinking and the headache is similar to the time it takes people to become flushed after alcohol. Roughly fifty per cent of sufferers know that alcohol provokes their attacks so they 'avoid it like the plague'. This sensitivity has its uses: when a cluster seems to be ending sufferers often employ what they call 'the alcohol test'. They take a small amount of alcohol to see if it produces a mild attack; when it does not, they start coming off their treatment.

Treatment

Sufferers often despair of ever being diagnosed, let alone finding effective treatment. However, for cluster headaches treatment works, and seven out of ten attacks can be stopped completely.

Abortive therapy: to stop an acute attack

Inhaling oxygen from a cylinder at a rate of seven litres per minute, using a firm plastic mask, can abort attacks within five to ten minutes. This method works for about six out of ten patients. The oxygen cylinder should be kept by the bedside so that as attacks begin the oxygen can be inhaled. The severe pains that normally last an hour should go within five to ten minutes. Having the correct mask is important. A large oxygen cylinder is usually needed, because the oxygen flow rate must be seven litres a minute (small cylinders manage only four litres a minute). General practitioners working within the National Health Service are able to prescribe oxygen for cluster headaches.

Prophylactic therapy

More effective than aborting attacks is to prevent them. Ergotamine tartrate is the most useful drug for this, although it is very powerful and must be used with care. Because arterial spasm is a possible side-effect, people with high blood pressure or arterial disease (which includes coronary artery disease) should avoid ergotamine (see page 121).

One effective way of taking ergotamine is in suppository form. If the attacks are happening at night (the usual time for cluster headaches), suppository should be inserted before going to bed. If attacks occur during the day, a suppository should be inserted in the morning.

After a few nights of freedom, the dosage can usually be reduced by cutting off a portion of the suppository so that only three-quarters, two-thirds, and eventually one-half is being used. As with any drug the minimum effective dose should be taken.

The second approach is to inhale ergotamine using a 'Medihaler', an aerosol preparation and inhaler. Four 'puffs' on retiring to bed should be effective initially, after which the dose can be progressively decreased. Most people have no side-effects from ergotamine, and when used for six to eight weeks, about as long as a cluster lasts, it is highly effective.

If ergotamine provides no relief or does so only with unacceptable side-effects, alternatives are available. Methysergide is very effective and safe for clusters of average duration. *Used for longer than five months it may have serious side-effects.* Some doctors have recommended that after five months' treatment there should be a drug-free interval of at least a month to minimise the risk of complications. Once again, the initial starting dose should be tailed off as the attacks become less severe. If methysergide fails, then there are other drugs available, such as pizotifen, prednisolone and lithium.

Chronic cluster headache

Finally, a rarity: occasionally the cluster does not end after eight weeks, but continues for many months. This condition, which is difficult to treat, was described only in 1976 by a Californian doctor (Dr Kudrow), who himself experiences cluster headaches. He has given a description of them in his book on this subject, *Cluster Headaches Mechanism & Management*, which is worthwhile reading for those affected.

CHAPTER 14

RESEARCH INTO MIGRAINES

THIS CHAPTER is divided into three parts. The first details the research on which this book is based. The second part describes some of the recent advances that have been made to increase our understanding of migraines and their treatment. Some of the research techniques that have led to progress are also given in this section. And finally, in the third part, some of the directions that current research is taking and future research needs to take are sketched out. But, first, a word about research in general.

Research in general

Research requires good ideas and persistence; sudden breakthroughs are rare. Even when what looks like a rapid advance has been made, many years of hard work will have preceded it (see page 124 for how long a new drug takes to reach the market). And breakthroughs often turn out to be illusory. Researchers may have made over-enthusiastic claims based on findings from small surveys or from pilot experiments. At least as often nowadays, however, it is the media, hungry for news, who have over-inflated the findings. Possible advances, quite soberly reported at medical conferences or in medical journals, get exaggerated almost out of recognition in the never-ending search for news. How many 'cancer cures', for example, have we heard about in the past decade?

Science progresses by research workers putting their ideas forward, and others attempting to confirm or refute them. Most suggestions do not stand the test of time. If they do, they may form the basis for new ideas, which are once again tested.

It is just as important to rid ourselves of mistaken beliefs that hinder progress, to refute wrong hypotheses, as it is to put forward new notions. Above all, rigorously controlled trials must be conducted on a sufficient number of people to provide meaningful answers.

Research on triggers for migraine attacks

Cheese and chocolate

Some 25 years ago Dr Edda Hanington noted that patients taking monoamine oxidase inhibitors (drugs used to treat depression) could develop sudden, severe headaches after eating cheese. This was explained by the drug's action on special enzymes, which led to increased levels of certain chemicals in the bloodstream after eating cheese. These circulated to the brain, causing the headaches.

Could the accumulation of the same chemicals explain the headaches of people who seemed sensitive to cheese? She asked 500 people who suffered from migraines which foods they avoided in the belief that they provoked migraines, and the proportions were as follows:

Chocolate (74%)

Cheese and dairy products (47%)

Fruit, particularly citrus fruits (30%)

Alcohol (18%)

Fried fatty foods (18%)

Vegetables (18%)

Tea or coffee (15%)

Meat, particularly pork (14%)

Seafood (10%).

Delving further into the problem she found her migraine patients more often avoided strong cheeses, such as Stilton and other blue cheeses, than simple cheeses like cottage cheese. She therefore postulated that a substance called tyramine, present in cheese, was responsible. Dr Hanington experimented by giving migraine sufferers either tyramine or a placebo (a dummy tablet) containing the sugar, lactose. Tyramine caused more migraines than the placebo, a fact which supported her hypothesis.

But there were problems – as can be seen from her results, her patients more often incriminated chocolate than cheese and dairy products – and chocolate contains no tyramine. Further research showed that other amines, phenylethylamine in chocolate and octopamine in citrus fruits, were the likely cause of migraines. Other research groups have tried repeating her studies, but not all of them agree with her findings.

Fasting and hypoglycaemia (low blood sugar)

In a study of the effects of fasting on migraines, two patients and ten volunteers – all of whom had migraines – were asked to stop eating after 10pm one evening. The next day they were allowed to drink only fluids, such as water, or tea or coffee without milk or sugar. Six of the twelve subjects developed their particular migraine while they were fasting. In five, their symptoms began between 9am and 12 noon, reaching their peak between 2pm and 7pm. The sixth subject's attack began at 7pm; she had fasted until 5pm when she rushed to collect her child from a nursery. On the way there, she stopped at a dairy where she drank half a pint of milk and ate some sweets. She collected her child, went home, and by 7pm her migraine had begun. It became a severe attack within two hours and lasted well into the night.

These findings were published in the *British Medical Journal*, and were reported a few days later by the *Daily Mirror*. A reader then wrote to the doctors who had conducted the study saying that his migraines had disappeared at the same time as he was diagnosed as suffering from diabetes.

This new observation, made by a patient, led to further research. An advertisement was placed in *Balance*, the journal of the British Diabetic Association, asking for any information from diabetic patients who were either suffering from migraine or had done so in the past. Thirty-six people with genuine migraines replied. Five patients had lost their migraines with the onset or control of diabetes and, in four other cases, migraines were precipitated when they had had too much insulin or insufficient food. This fitted closely with the theory that fasting provoked migraines. Food deprivation and insulin lower the blood glucose; in diabetes, blood glucose is raised.

This observation has since been confirmed in a much larger study of headaches in diabetics and non-diabetics. The results showed that those with diabetes had fewer headaches and migraine attacks than people without diabetes and that insulin can precipitate migraine attacks in six out of eleven insulin-dependent diabetics who also had other triggers.

Blood glucose therefore seems to be important in headaches in general and in migraines in particular. Children and sportsmen and women seem particularly prone to fasting-induced migraine – their attacks may be relieved by eating food or taking pure glucose. More importantly, eating an adequate breakfast or a lunch can prevent migraines, avoiding the need to take medication – either abortive or prophylactic.

CASE HISTORY

When the Soviet dissident Anatoly Shcharansky, stopped his hunger strike, he telephoned his mother to say that he was feeling better and his headache was beginning to disappear.

Female hormones

Dr Ellen Grant, who worked in a family planning clinic, found that some of her patients noticed that their migraines increased whilst they were taking the oral contraceptive pill. Some of these women needed to have a D & C (dilatation and curettage) operation of the uterus. Examining the specimens under a microscope revealed that patients who suffered from migraines had more blood vessels lining the womb than women without headaches. This suggested to her that the hormones contained in the pill had a direct effect on the blood vessels in the lining of the womb. From this Dr Grant inferred that the pill may also have direct effects on blood vessels in the brain, and evidence for this has been found.

Eyes

Several different research groups have studied visual stimulation and migraines. One group found that when patients were subjected to certain patterns where lines are close to each other for 30 seconds or longer, one-sided headaches were likely to occur. The group also noticed that some people with a migraine have abnormalities of the electrical impulses in the brain.

Some migraine sufferers have found for themselves that certain patterns can give rise to headaches if looked at long enough. Tension headaches and migraines are being frequently reported by the operators of VDUs. Not all screens are the same, however – their backgrounds may differ, as may the colour of the text. More studies are needed to tease out the main problem or problems. Further research will have to make allowances for the variations that exist among people – some are more sensitive to noise, others to light. The findings from one specially selected group of people may therefore not necessarily apply to everyone. Research that on first sight looks easy to do and interpret often proves to be very difficult.

Recently it has been shown that fluorescent lighting is of two types: flickering and non-flickering. The flickering variety gives rise to EEG changes – the brain waves of those prone to headaches are shown to be more changeable than those not subject to headaches. If substantiated, these findings have important implications for the way lighting is used in shops, large stores, as well as in the home.

A novel idea comes from the Hammersmith Hospital, London where a young doctor has produced goggles which shine flickering lights at migraine sufferers. Preliminary results indicate that migraine attacks can be stopped in half an hour. The goggles also seem useful in preventing attacks, perhaps by de-conditioning the sufferers.

The dental approach

There is no doubt that dental problems can cause pain on one or both sides of the head. Usually this is due to malocclusion, where the teeth on one side are higher than the other, resulting in an asymmetrical 'bite'. Correcting this abnormality may relieve the headaches.

The British Migraine Association arranged for 20 patients with migraines from the Charing Cross Hospital Migraine Clinic to be seen by a professor of dental surgery at Guy's Hospital Dental School who was particularly interested in dental malocclusion. He found that six of the 20 had abnormalities of bite, which was then corrected. One of the six reported fewer migraines. If this were a representative sample, and with such small numbers it is difficult to be sure, then perhaps one in 20 migraine sufferers could be helped in this way.

Pain can arise in the jaw joint of the masticatory muscles, especially the temporal muscle on one side of the head. This pain can trigger migraine attacks but the pain itself may be mistaken for a migraine, because it is one-sided.

The neck and migraine

Problems with the neck may cause headaches, and the pain can be referred to the forehead or the eyes. This is due to a very peculiar arrangement of the nerve supply; operations carried out under local anaesthesia have shown that stimulating the nerves of the upper neck can be felt as pain in the forehead.

This may explain how physiotherapy, chiropractic, acupuncture or osteopathy concentrating on the neck can in *some* people relieve their migraine trigger.

A problem which has not been tackled so far is that some people during their migraine attacks feel that their neck is stiff. In fact, it may be a warning symptom: neck stiffness may be noticed even before the headache begins. Such a stiffening was recorded by the late Belgian physician Dr Jan Waelkens who found that his patients complained of their necks feeling tight or 'short', making it difficult for them to bend forward hours before their headaches began.

Another symptom that is not fully understood is pain on the surface of the head during a migraine attack. The pain arises in the superficial muscles, which may remain tender to touch for a day or two after the headache has gone. It may be that these muscles go into spasm, having been overactive during the headache, leaving the sort of muscle pain that is felt after over-exertion (similar to the muscle contraction headaches described on page 32).

The weather and migraine

Some migraine sufferers are convinced that their attacks occur when the barometric pressure changes, particularly when there is thundery weather about. Research from Israel supports their hunch. A professor there has identified a group of migraine sufferers whose attacks seem to be triggered by sudden changes of weather.

A study at the City of London Migraine Clinic, however, failed to confirm these findings. Researchers could find no relationship between the frequency of attacks and changes of temperature and barometric pressure recorded by the observatory at Kew Gardens. The negative finding does not necessarily mean that the hypothesis is wrong. It may be that weather changes in England are not as sudden or as exceptional as they are in the Middle East.

An association between climate and disease is not a new notion. It is well known that conditions such as heart attacks and stomach ulcers are more likely to occur at certain times of the year.

Recent advances

We can be optimistic about the next 25 years, bearing in mind the progress made in the understanding and treatment of migraine during the past quarter of a century. Here are some of these advances.

The attitude of the medical profession

Many more doctors are now interested in migraine and other headaches than ever were in the past. They are prepared to admit that there is no cure, and that they do not know the cause of migraine. Much more research is now being carried out, both in migraine clinics and in laboratories. Researchers have stopped labelling the condition as 'psychosomatic', an unkind label, serving only to hinder further enquiry. Admitting that psychological factors may be important is one thing but to maintain that migraine is 'all in the mind' is untrue, unhelpful to the patient, and not constructive for future research.

What has made doctors become more interested? One important factor may have been the increased interest shown in migraines by the public. The greatest stimulus to research comes from questioning.

Lay interest in migraine

In Britain, migraine sufferers formed an organisation, the British Migraine Association in 1962 (see page 169 for address). Since then, similar groups have been set up in many other countries. These have exerted gentle but firm pressure on the medical profession to look deeper into the problem. These groups, consisting mostly of sufferers and their relatives, have made it clear that they want to know more. So they ask questions. They raise money to fund research into the cause and treatment of migraine. The British Migraine Association, for example, with more than 8,000 members, answers enquiries from members and funds research projects; it publishes a quarterly newsletter which contains vigorous correspondence. The American National Headache Foundation is a larger body which also has a newsletter, supports research and runs courses for general practitioners and specialist physicians interested in migraine.

Communication among doctors

The Migraine Trust (see page 169 for address) started supporting treatment and research into migraine in 1966. Similar societies are now flourishing in many countries. As a result, clinics especially for people suffering from migraines and headaches have opened in Britain, the United States, Canada, Ireland, Australia and New Zealand. In 1983 the International Headache Society was formed, which has become the largest headache organisation in the world. At its most recent international conference there were more than 900 participants from 30 countries.

Conferences are useful for doctors and research scientists to share their findings and discuss common problems. They cost large sums of money, however, usually donated by drug companies and research organisations. The formal part of the conference revolves around the presentation of papers reporting experimental observations and investigations, including drug trials. Just as important is what happens outside these formal sessions when interested parties can get together and swap their ideas and experiences informally.

Conferences are reported in the organising society's journal or are gathered together in a book once the authors have had time to reconsider the papers they presented at the conference, often modified in the light of their own and others' criticisms. Two journals are devoted purely to headache. One is suitably called *Headache*, published by the American Association for the Study of Headache; the other is entitled *Cephalalgia*, which has become the official journal of the International Headache Society. In addition, wide-circulation, general medical journals, such as the *British Medical Journal*, *The Lancet*, *Journal of the American Medical Association*, and the *New England Journal of Medicine*, keep their readers up to date with headache research and are publishing more original papers on headaches and migraines.

Observations on patients

There is continuing research on the effects of migraine on sufferers. The opening of the Migraine Clinic in the City of London in 1971 was a major advance in itself, and has led to other advances. At the clinic, migraine sufferers can be seen not only between attacks but *during* attacks. The importance of this for the understanding of migraines cannot be overestimated.

From observations at the City Clinic, the various phases of a migraine attack have been delineated, as has the importance of sleep in ending attacks. A new kind of headache due to overdosage of ergotamine tartrate (which is used to treat migraines) was first described by Dr Marcia Wilkinson of the City Clinic.

Another new headache, due to insufficient sleep, has recently been reported (August 1990): it is not a 'tension headache' as formerly believed and responds well to two (or even one) analgesic tablets.

Work on what triggers migraine is being done in several places. The finding that the oral contraceptive pill made migraines worse has stimulated reinvestigation of menstrual migraine showing that it is important in *some* women.

Recent population studies have shown that migraine is universal, and that headaches and migraines are more common than was previously thought. Women with migraine attacks seem to have fewer strokes and less coronary disease than their counterparts who do not have migraines – a surprise to the investigators and others.

In diabetics the incidence of headache and migraine is less than in people without diabetes, implying that a high blood sugar may protect against headache while a low blood sugar increases the risk.

Drug studies

Metoclopramide has been found to be very useful in migraines because it accelerates stomach emptying. Migraines delay drug absorption in the gut: by giving metoclopramide early in the attack its effect on stomach emptying helps to improve the absorption of other drugs, for example, analgesics. As a result metoclopramide is now included in some proprietary preparations.

In the past decade ways of measuring blood levels of ergotamine using a radioisotope immune assay have been devised. Tests on people taking the drug have shown that some cannot absorb ergotamine when it is taken by mouth, which explains why a proportion of sufferers find the drug has no effect.

Certain amines have been found in foods – including tyramine in cheese, phenylethylamine in chocolate, and octopamine in citrus fruits (see page 135). Other amines that act on the blood vessels may be present in various wines or citrus fruits. These could be responsible for the migraine attacks that some people experience after ingesting them.

Not having the right enzymes to detoxify certain chemicals may be to blame for some people's migraine. Attacks following red wine may be due to the absence of the enzyme phenolsulphotransferase, which deactivates phenols. More research is being done on some of the body's own chemicals that constrict and dilate blood vessels, such as 5-hydroxytryptamine and prostaglandins.

Much research has been done on food allergy as a possible cause of migraines. In people whose attacks seem to be related to food, sodium cromoglycate, an anti-allergic drug used in asthma, has been useful.

Certain neurotransmitters, the chemicals that convey messages from one nerve cell to another, such as dopamine, enkephalins, endorphins and especially 5-hydroxytryptamine, are being vigorously investigated to see whether they have a primary role in migraines.

Techniques and topics of research

Measuring cerebral blood flow

The Scandinavian work described on page 100 gives a good idea of the value of this technique. These procedures were first tested on animals to reduce the risk to man.

PET scanning

In the last few years, a new method of assessing the brain's metabolism has been introduced, using Positron Emission Tomography (PET). In this technique a small dose of radioactive oxygen or glucose, introduced into the circulation, can be measured in various parts of the brain. The preliminary results suggest that there is less oxygen and glucose taken up by the brain during a migraine attack. This is in keeping with the findings of cerebral blood flow measurements. It is more exciting than that, however, because eventually researchers should be able to localise exactly where this reduction occurs. It is possible, in the next few years, being able to say exactly which parts of the brain are affected during attacks.

Magneto-encephalography and brain spectro-photometry

These two techniques were first reported in 1989 in the USA. One uses a very powerful magnet to study variations in the brain during migraine. The other detects chemical variations: this indicates that magnesium levels may be altered in migraine.

Neuroendocrinology

The 1980s have witnessed major advances in neurochemistry and neuroendocrinology. The latter is particularly concerned with a part of the brain called the hypothalamus, which controls the involuntary nervous system and the pituitary gland.

Neurotransmitters, chemicals by which nerves communicate with each other, have been the focus of intensive research recently. Some are concerned with sending messages; others with amplifying, modulating or inhibiting nerve impulses. Obviously crucial to the functioning of the brain, neurotransmitters also seem to be important in headaches.

Nerve control of blood vessels

Another large area of research concerns how nerves control the diameter of blood vessels. A group in Boston, USA, has focused on substance P, a chemical concerned with pain, and shown that the trigeminal ganglion in the head, which transmits sensations (including pain) from the head, influences not only meningeal vessels on the surface of the brain but also extends to the face. Before researchers can study what is abnormal, they must know the normal control mechanisms first and, with new fluorescent stains, these nerves are now being accurately mapped.

Pineal gland

The importance of the pineal gland (called the third eye in the past) has recently been recognised, though its function remains unclear. It produces a substance called melatonin, which may regulate the body's circadian rhythm (that is, the regular pattern of going to sleep once a day and feeling hungry two or three times a day). Melatonin has recently been tried in air-crews to prevent jet-lag. A study from Oslo has shown that the melatonin in the blood increases more in people with cluster headaches than in those without. Whether these are linked as cause and effect is not yet known.

Psychological approaches

Much work has been done on behaviour and personality, and treatments stemming from this work – such as biofeedback – have been used in migraine and headache clinics, particularly in the United States. Personality cannot be a full explanation, however: in clinical practice many well-balanced people who do not seem to be under stress suffer from migraine.

Visual approaches

It is well known that flashing lights can provoke migraine. Some years ago a technique to measure how the back of the brain responded when the eyes were stimulated by flashing lights was introduced into neurology. In migraine sufferers *between* attacks, this response is delayed. So what happens during attacks? Finding out is difficult: not only does the person have a severe headache, but he or she also wants to avoid bright lights.

In the late 1980s, a group in Birmingham found changes in the visual evoked potentials (EEG changes produced by flashing lights recorded from the back of the brain). These are found more in visual migraine and in classical, as distinct from common, migraines and are also more evident in children.

These observations are being repeated in other laboratories: the results are eagerly awaited because they could provide the first diagnostic test for migraine.

The future

There are certain goals towards which doctors are currently striving:

- A specific test for migraine, biological or biochemical, which allows them to say whether or not someone suffers from migraine.
- More effective preventive therapy: currently, the best drugs have only a 60 per cent efficacy and it is impossible to predict who the unlucky 40 per cent of sufferers are.
- More effective drugs to abort attacks: aiming for 100 per cent effective control may be unrealistic – the best that may be possible is to convert a migraine into an ordinary headache, lasting two to four hours rather than a whole day.
- More research into headaches other than migraines. This could contribute towards a greater understanding of migraines themselves.
- More research into biochemistry, pharmacology and the relatively new sciences of neurochemistry and neuroendocrinology.
- More clinical studies of people during attacks of migraine. This is not easy, particularly when they are vomiting or in severe pain. Many people, however, whose headaches are

mild or only moderately severe could co-operate in some of the research that needs to be conducted.

Overall, medical researchers are hopeful and confident about the future. Certainly, judging by recent advances and the speed at which progress is accelerating, further increases in knowledge can be expected.

CHAPTER **15**

MIGRAINE AND HEADACHE CLINICS

PATIENT satisfaction provides the strongest justification for the existence of specialised clinics. The second justification is research. Special migraine or headache clinics have now sprung up all over the world; these may be self-contained or linked to the neurological department of a hospital.

They were pioneered by Dr Macdonald Critchley, a London neurologist, who in 1955 started a special weekly outpatient clinic for migraine sufferers. Appointments were made between 5 and 7pm so that patients did not lose time from work. A few other neurological departments copied this model.

In 1971, at the instigation of the husband of a migraine sufferer, a new approach was tried. The first clinic in the world where patients could be treated *during* attacks opened in the City of London. In the first four years, 2,000 patients received treatment while in the throes of an acute headache – mostly migraines but also some with acute tension headache. A further 6,000 patients attended for consultations *between* attacks. Such numbers demanded larger premises and the Clinic moved to Charterhouse Square, London EC1.

The City of London Migraine Clinic is now world famous and although most patients come from or near London, others come from much further afield. Doctors from foreign countries visit or work at the Clinic, which not only treats patients but also conducts research.

Some of the research described in this book originated from the Clinic: for example, the benefit of combining an anti-nausea drug with an ordinary analgesic in the treatment of an acute attack (page 118) and the first proper scientific trial of the effect of feverfew in preventing headaches. Premonitory symptoms (page 76) and migraines were studied for the first time at the Clinic.

Advice is also sought by pharmaceutical companies on drug trials of new preparations.

The knowledge acquired has been disseminated in Britain to occupational nurses and doctors, general practitioners and hospital doctors. A measure of success is that fewer people now attend the clinic during acute attacks than in its early days – they are now being treated successfully at work, thanks to the local educational initiative.

The Clinic is a registered medical charity and all the consultants give their time and services for free. Patients are not charged but can, if they wish, make a donation towards the upkeep of the clinic and towards research. The Clinic is supported by the British Migraine Association, the City, industry and other donors.

What benefits does the patient derive from a specialised clinic?

The person who attends during an attack is taken to a darkened room, seen by the clinic's nursing sister and a doctor, and then treated immediately rather than perhaps waiting in a casualty department where people with coronaries or severe injuries, naturally, are treated first. For people working in the City of London such immediate care and attention is preferable to travelling home by public transport struggling with nausea and headache.

People who come for consultations between attacks benefit from the skill of the staff who know migraine's uncommon manifestations, rare complications and unusual precipitating factors. Sufferers rapidly sense that they have found a doctor who knows all about their migraines and is interested by them.

In addition to the City of London Migraine Clinic being used as a model in establishing further migraine clinics in London (see page 169 for addresses), its success has led to the development of clinics in North America, Scandinavia and other European countries.

Aside from caring for patients, migraine clinics provide valuable research potential for doctors specialising in headaches and migraines.

All in all, research into and treatment for migraines and headaches is flourishing. It needs to grow more, to increase our understanding and knowledge of the conditions and enable better treatment to be given.

APPENDIX

COMPLEMENTARY THERAPIES

What is complementary medicine?

COMPLEMENTARY medicine differs in approach from allopathy (conventional drug treatment) in that it promotes self-healing, sometimes, in the case of homoeopathy, by mimicking the symptoms it intends to cure.

Alternative medicine is not a strictly accurate term, as many alternative practitioners maintain that what they do is not to seek to replace orthodox medicine but to enhance it by working alongside it. Reputable practitioners would not consider trying to treat a patient with an illness requiring surgery, for example; instead they may work closely with the patient and provide relaxation techniques to aid and stimulate recovery.

Headaches, as previously discussed, very rarely require surgery (see chapter 4 for those that do), and are considered by complementary therapists to be highly suitable for their type of treatment. Indeed, those migraines and headaches that are stress-related may be treated beneficially by the treatments described below.

Complementary therapists may view the individual illness as something that affects the whole person and not the particular organ or part of the body that is actually suffering. They therefore treat the whole person in response. Practitioners ask a series of very varied questions about a person's lifestyle, diet, work, relaxation, state of mind, etc., so that they can build up a complete picture. The cause of someone's headache will not always be obvious. In many therapies, once the cause of the headache has been established, there is no one precise form of treatment: in homoeopathy (see page 161) and aromatherapy (see page 158) treatment is tailored to meet the individual's 'personality needs' as well as confronting the headache or migraine symptoms.

The availability of complementary medicine

Access to complementary medicine is still very patchy: there are more practitioners in the south of England than in the rest of the UK. More GPs, however, are now willing to refer patients to complementary practitioners then ever before; and many more now additionally provide complementary therapies themselves. If you go to a complementary therapist and find that his or her approach does not suit you, it does not necessarily mean that a certain therapy is not for you. Do not dismiss the therapy out of hand, but persevere and visit another practitioner whose methods and personality may suit you better.

What to expect

As has been stated, complementary medicine treats the whole person and therefore when someone is referred by a GP, or approaches a lay practitioner, the therapist will require a very detailed medical and life history★. The person will be questioned on what may seem to be unrelated points about his or her health, state of mind, career prospects, family life, and so on, so that the practitioner can build a detailed picture. Questioning may also be supplemented by X-rays and routine medical tests.

There may well be some immediate relief gained from the therapy, or progress over a period of time; but, in some cases, an actual initial slight worsening of the condition may mean that the treatment is taking effect.

Complementary therapies will draw a person's attention to the stresses of the mind and body and may initiate the body's self-healing processes. Even if treatment cannot help prevent headaches or migraines, there may well be a lessening of attacks in both frequency and severity, as well as encouraging a feeling of well-being.

★ This also applies to orthodox medicine. See pages 68-70.

Regulatory control

In Britain there are neither laws governing the practice of complementary medicine, nor any centralised training, so that anyone can set him or herself up as a lay practitioner without recourse to any single body.

Most complementary therapies, however, have their own representative bodies which provide guidelines regarding training, and will supply the general public with a list of therapists. Just because complementary therapies tend to use natural products in their healing, that is not an indication that they are any safer than conventional drugs, especially in inexperienced hands. See pages 173-5 for addresses of some representative bodies concerned with complementary medicine.

Practitioners can also charge what they like for treatment, so it is advisable to find out beforehand how much a practitioner will charge for a consultation, each session and the number of sessions that will be required.

Acupuncture

Acupuncture is an ancient Chinese art dating from several thousand years ago. Chinese philosophy maintains that there is a vital essence or life, known as *chi*, which is composed of *yin* and *yang* (negative and positive) elements, and that the imbalance of *yin* and *yang*, which causes disharmony in body and mind, can be corrected by acupuncture.

What is acupuncture?

The word acupuncture is derived from the Latin words *acus* (needle) and *punctura* (to prick). Certain strategic points on the body are pierced with fine stainless steel needles and may be stimulated with massage, heat or electricity. Relief can occur in areas close to the needles and/or in distant areas of the body.

Acupuncture is based on the nervous connection between the body's organs and its surface. When an organ is diseased, pain may be referred to points on, or just under, the skin. Stimulation of these and other non-tender acupuncture points sends impulses to the central nervous system and so influences the corresponding area of the body.

The Chinese describe about 1,000 acupuncture points which are divided into twelve groups, joined by imaginary lines on the surface of the body called meridians, each associated with different areas or organs of the body.

The diagnosis

In traditional Chinese medicine, diagnosis was based on a history of the person's health and observation and examination of the tongue, confirmed by an elaborate pulse diagnosis. Nowadays, the acupuncturist follows much the same approach as any conventional physician, taking a full medical history followed by a detailed medical examination.

Having made a diagnosis, the acupuncturist chooses the appropriate treatment for the complaint. The acupuncturist must use his or her clinical judgement to decide whether acupuncture can relieve the condition or whether, in extreme cases, it is serious enough to warrant surgery.

How is it done?

The acupuncture points are stimulated with disposable or sterilised needles. The needles are inserted to various depths in the skin. Sometimes, an electrical current is passed down a needle or the points are stimulated via surface electrodes, laser, heat or massage.

In manual acupuncture, the skilled acupuncturist decides on the gauge of the needle, how to manipulate it, how deep to insert it, how long to leave it in place, and the frequency and number of treatments. Different needle manipulations, and varying frequencies of electrical stimulation, have different therapeutic effects.

What does the person experience?

Treatment is normally painless; however, there might be a slight 'needling sensation' known as *t'chi*, which is a heavy dull feeling. Indeed, when this occurs it is often an indication of a positive response. Response times vary: sometimes relief is immediate; sometimes there will be an improvement over a number of days or weeks and sometimes there will be no response at all.

A sense of well-being and relaxation is very common. Therefore, acupuncture is a helpful medium in relieving the body of stress, the major cause of headaches. Sometimes a temporary exacerbation of the condition may occur but this almost always happens with the first treatment and may predict an eventually successful outcome.

How does it work?

The insertion of needles produces pain-relieving effects by stimulating neurochemical mediators (endorphins) found naturally within the brain. These endorphins are produced at different rates in response to the body's requirements and are used to combat the pain of headaches. The stimulation increases their production and the sensation of pain is lessened.

Many GPs refer patients they think would benefit from this treatment to a registered acupuncturist. Medically qualified acupuncturists are accountable to the General Medical Council and have professional indemnity insurance.

There is no licensing body for acupuncture. The public can receive a list of registered medical practitioners from the British Medical Acupuncture Association. For the address see page 173.

Alexander Technique

The Alexander Technique was developed in the nineteenth century by the Australian actor Frederick Matthias Alexander. Alexander was prompted to find a solution to his recurring problem of losing his voice when public speaking. He discovered that he was misusing his body, which in turn affected his breathing and his voice, and from this diagnosis he formulated the technique named after him, which he began teaching in 1894.

How does it work?

The Technique involves changing bad postural habits, and taking a fresh look at the way a person thinks and moves. Excessive effort and tension on spinal muscles develop from early childhood and cause problems which are exacerbated as the years pass. It is necessary for the student of the Alexander Technique to relearn more appropriate habits that promote better functioning of the spinal area. The stresses on the spine attributed to bad posture affect the muscles and nerves in the back and neck, which can lead to headaches and migraines. The Alexander Technique allows the spine to lengthen and the strains to dissipate.

In an Alexander Technique lesson a 'teacher' may make physical adjustments to a 'pupil's' body by oral instruction and by using his or her hands. A pupil may be asked to sit down, lie down, adopt a standing posture or walk around, while developing the awareness to recognise and release unnecessary tension and effort. The new postures adopted may initially feel very strange if they are different from long-standing habits. Therefore, the technique needs to be practised until fluency is achieved. The whole learning experience can be regarded as more a mental exercise than a physical one. There is as much emphasis on an awareness of a pupil's state of mind as on movement and manipulation.

A pupil may need anything from 10 to 30 lessons (or more) to achieve an improvement. Initial success is very difficult to detect.

Specialist teachers undergo a three-year training programme under the auspices of The Society of Teachers of the Alexander Technique. Alexander Technique teachers should hold a certificate of authority issued by the Society. Further details can be received from the Society by sending a 9″ × 6″ s.a.e. to the address on page 173.

Aromatherapy

Aromatherapy is an ancient holistic treatment which aromatherapists believe helps restore the body's natural rhythm and so enables self-healing processes to begin. Aromatherapy can be useful in the treatment of headaches and migraines by relieving stressful symptoms. The aromatherapist utilises essential oils, which are pure aromatic essences extracted or distilled from a variety of natural products such as flowers, trees, herbs and fruit. These oils are then blended with pure vegetable oils and are massaged, by various means, into the skin. The oils are absorbed into the bloodstream and are transmitted throughout the body. The temperature at which the aromatics are applied is crucial: body temperature is ideal for absorption and a warm compress may be used by a practitioner to aid penetration. Massage is an important part of the process as it can help locate the stressful points on the body that require more treatment.

There are about 60 main oils in use, each with its own unique properties. Some of the oils used by aromatherapists include chamomile, grapefruit, lavender, peppermint and rosemary. Each formula is prepared individually for the person concerned after a very detailed life and medical history has been taken by the aromatherapist, looking at diet, stress, exercise and allergy factors.

The International Federation of Aromatherapists is a representative, but not a licensing, body for aromatherapists. To receive a list of registered members send an s.a.e. to the address on page 173.

Biofeedback

Feedback is a natural occurrence: when our bodies cannot do something, for instance, heavy lifting, they protest with pain as a warning. This involuntary feedback is mimicked in biofeedback.

The process began as a laboratory technique. It is useful in headaches and migraines because it teaches the individual how to relax and to avoid stress. Biofeedback machines measure a variety of natural processes: blood pressure, heart rate and muscle tension. In biofeedback treatment a person is connected to an electrical device that delivers an audio-visual signal directly related to activity in the scalp and in the hand. The machine may measure the contraction of scalp muscles and also sweat and temperature readings from the hands. A rise in temperature, for example, means that the person is relaxing.

Thought processes can be used to regulate the visual or audio pulses on the biofeedback machine. After some experience, a person learns to affect and eventually control his or her blood flow to the skin, muscle tension or heart rate. Success comes when the person is able to duplicate at will the thought processes leading to this control. Reducing muscle tension helps relieve the effects of tension headaches.

For further details about biofeedback ask your GP.

Chiropractic

Chiropractic – *cheiro* (hand) and *practikos* (practice) – was developed in the 1890s in the USA by Daniel David Palmer. His research revealed that if there was a disturbance in the function of spinal joints and muscles there would be a corresponding impaired function of the nervous system. In headaches and migraines stiffness in the spinal joints can cause neck muscle tension and lead to head pain. It takes only a minor spinal displacement or *subluxation*, as it is known to chiropractics, to irritate a nerve supply, leading to body malfunction and disease.

Chiropractic is similar to osteopathy (see page 164), but differs from it in the diagnosis and method of treatment. Osteopaths treat joints in order to improve mobility; relief of a certain condition is achieved by working on muscles and tendons using leverage and applying pressure to shoulders and hips. Chiropractors unlock stiff joints and use short, high velocity and shallow thrusts on the point of subluxation. The chiropractor has about 40 different adjustment techniques at his or her disposal. Relief may be achieved after only one visit to a therapist or a series of consultations may be necessary.

A practitioner will take a detailed personal medical history and possibly also X-rays and routine medical tests to decide whether a person is suffering from a disease or injury where it would be unwise to use chiropractic techniques and where orthodox medicine is more appropriate.

Benefits may be immediate or long-term. As well as helping

to lessen the frequency and severity of headaches, chiropractic can also benefit the body as a whole. Chiropractors may also use massage and are keen to promote muscle re-education and remedy postural faults.

Chiropractors who have taken a four-year course can become members of the British Chiropractors Association. Names of qualified chiropractors on the register can be obtained by writing to the Association at the address given on page 173.

Homoeopathy

The word homoeopathy is derived from the Greek words *homoios* (similar) and *pathos* (suffering). Homoeopathy was established in Europe in the nineteenth century by the German physician Samuel Hahnemann who was dissatisfied with medical practice at the time, considering it brutal and inhumane. He resolved that the approach to medicine could be by more subtle means.

There are three major principles of homoeopathy:
- like cures like
- infinitesimal doses
- treatment of the person rather than the disease.

Like cures like

Homoeopaths regard disease as the healthy outward manifestation of the body's internal struggle. Homoeopathy takes a seemingly paradoxical approach. The challenge is not to reduce the disease but to encourage the body's own healing ability. The idea of homoeopathy can be compared to the vaccination process, in which a minute dose of a disease is actually given to combat it. In homoeopathy a minute dose of a medicine that in a healthy person would produce symptoms of the illness stimulates the body's healing process. There may well be a slight worsening of the condition before there is an improvement. This can signify that the healing has begun.

Infinitesimal doses

The remedies, as in other complementary therapies, are tailored to meet individual requirements, so a detailed diagnosis and history of the person will be drawn up by the practitioner. All the remedies are prepared from pure animal, vegetable and mineral sources. Minute doses are prescribed: these are repeatedly shaken and diluted (a process known as potentisation). At each stage of the process, one drop of the ingredient is mixed with 99 drops of water, and shaken until the final concentration is less than one millionth part of the original solution, or mother tincture, as it is known. Paradoxically, homoeopathic remedies are stronger the more dilute they are.

Treatment of the person rather than the disease

A variety of substances, over 3,000 in total, are used by homoeopaths. Some of the homoeopathic remedies used for headache include Belladonna, Ignatia, Natrum muriaticum, Kali bichronicum and Silicea. The remedies are designed to fit the personality and not the disease so homoeopathic practitioners may need to try several remedies before a correct match is found for an individual. Three people may all complain of headaches, yet the treatment will be different for each one.

Homoeopathic treatment is available on the National Health Service. There are at present five homoeopathic hospitals (see page 174 for details). The British Homoeopathic Association (see page 173) provides a list of GPs (send an s.a.e.) who have had postgraduate homoeopathic training at the Faculty of Homoeopathy; they often have MFHom after their names. Lay homoeopaths are registered with the Society of Homoeopaths (see page 173) and have undergone four years' training, though none of the courses for lay practitioners has any legal recognition as yet.

Medical herbalism

The origins of medical herbalism date back many thousands of years and extend to very many different cultures. It is the most widely practised complementary therapy in the world. Evidence of its antiquity comes from a Chinese herbal dating from 2,500 BC which lists 365 herbs and ancient Egyptian papyri which list 700 plant medicines. *Gerards's Herbal*, printed in England in 1636, describes the medicinal uses of about 3,800 plants.

Like other complementary therapies, medical herbalism is geared towards treating the whole person and not the disease. Therefore, each remedy is tailored individually by taking into account the person's general health, diet, posture, exercise, stress levels, and so on. Herbalists will perform a physical examination and routine tests. Two entirely different remedies may be given to treat the same disease in two different people.

The allopathic approach to medicine, in finding, isolating and distilling the active principle from the plant, such as aspirin from willow bark and digoxin from foxglove, is rejected by herbal practitioners. Herbalists emphasise that these elements are taken out of context and that the plants in their natural state are 'in balance'. They would prefer to give an extract of the whole plant rather than elements from it. *Ma huang*, a Chinese herb, yields ephedrine – an alkaloid which results in high blood pressure if given as an extracted drug. However, one of the six other alkaloids in the plant actually has the reverse effect of lowering blood pressure, thereby combatting the potentially dangerous element in the herb.

Herbalism can be used to treat both immediate symptoms and long-term problems. The benefits someone may expect range from a reduction in frequency and severity of attacks to full prevention of recurrence; treatment is unlikely to be confined to the actual time of a migraine, but given over a period to restore balance and health. It is extremely unwise to self-administer herbal remedies; a qualified herbal practitioner's advice should be sought.

Plant medicines are most commonly prescribed in liquid form, as tinctures, fluids or syrups, but are also available as tablets, capsules, ointments and poultices.

Many current orthodox medicines were originally developed from herbal remedies and there has been considerable new research into the potential of this kind of medicine. There are over ¾ million species of plant still awaiting investigation.

More information can be obtained from the National Institute of Medical Herbalists. The address is on page 174.

Osteopathy

Osteopathy is a system of manual medicine which is concerned with the structural and mechanical problems of the body. It was founded by Doctor Andrew Taylor Still in the USA in the early 1870s. The aim of osteopathy is to restore proper function and mobility to the body's framework or musculoskeletal system by means of gentle passive stretching movements and specific manipulation of restricted joints.

When someone consults an osteopath, the osteopath will take a full and detailed case history. The osteopath will then conduct a careful examination, which will include orthodox medical, orthopaedic and neurological tests. A detailed structural assessment of the joints and their surrounding muscles and ligaments will also be carried out to see if they are functioning normally. At the end of this examination the osteopath will decide whether or not the person is likely to respond to osteopathic treatment.

In those people who are complaining of persistent headaches, osteopaths frequently find the head pain is accompanied by pain and stiffness in the neck and shoulders. If there has been a history of recent or severe injury, the osteopath may request that an X-ray is taken or ask for a report on any X-rays that have been taken previously. Frequently, in people who are suffering from persistent headaches, the small muscles at the base of the skull are very tight, contracted and tender to touch. Osteopathic treatment in such cases consists of gentle, manual pressure to the base of the skull to ease the muscular spasm, followed by gentle, rhythmical movements to stretch the tense and contracted tissues. If there are areas in the upper neck where the joints are stiff, these may be eased by specific mobilisation techniques. A treatment session usually lasts between 20 to 30 minutes.

Many tension headaches respond to treatment immediately, although long-standing problems may take several treatments. People suffering from headaches are often given advice on posture.

Registered osteopaths can be identified by the letters 'MRO' after their name and have all undergone a four-year full-time course of training at one of the three schools accredited by the General Council and Register of Osteopaths (GCRO). The GCRO provides an information service to members of the public and also publishes a Directory of Members which is available on request.

Reflexology

Reflexology is a pressure therapy applied to specific parts of the feet. Each zone or area of the foot correlates to the different parts of the body (arm, head, leg, etc.) and different organs. Massage and pressure on the soles of the feet are helpful in such stress-related disorders as headaches. Practitioners may also use zones on the hand in a similar manner. Like most other complementary therapies, reflexology is concerned with maintaining health and preventing illness, as well as being some help in relieving the pain of headaches.

The hands of the practitioner are essential in creating both dynamic and sensitive movements to relieve pain. If a person feels pain when a therapist is massaging a certain zone it reveals that there is a disturbance, pressure or blockage in the life flow there. Like other holistic treatments, reflexology is unsuitable in certain cases: conditions requiring surgery, infectious diseases, etc.

Self-treatment is difficult – the sensitivity of the hands of the practitioner is all-important.

More information can be received by writing to the British School of Reflexology, whose address appears on page 175.

Shiatsu

Shiatsu, the Japanese word meaning 'finger pressure', is a therapy based upon Oriental medicine. Shiatsu applies stretching and pressure throughout the body to the same energy channels (meridians) as used in acupuncture (see page 155). This pressure can be applied using fingers, thumbs, palms, elbows, knees and feet.

Apart from rebalancing the flow of energy within the channels, shiatsu also stimulates blood and lymphatic fluid circulation, helping to release waste products that have built up in the muscles, ease tension and generally aid relaxation.

According to Oriental medicine, imbalances in the 'liver' and 'gall bladder channels' are often the cause of migraines, and digestive imbalances can cause headaches. Traditionally, shiatsu is able to disperse the *Ki* (blocked energy) flow to the head and also regulate the *Ki* in the 'liver' and 'gall bladder'.

Shiatsu works in both the short and the long term. Gentle practice of shiatsu to the Gall Bladder channel to the side of the head could initially relieve symptoms. Further treatment on the back of the skull (known as area Gall Bladder 20) clears stagnant *Ki*. Fingertip pressure between the eyebrows is also beneficial.

Certain herbs, such a feverfew, skullcap, peppermint and red sage, and oils may be used to supplement treatment. Essential oils, containing lavender, chamomile and marjoram can also be applied and massaged into the meridians.

As with other holistic treatments, the easing of pain is combined with treating the underlying cause of imbalances, to enable the body to generate its own self-healing properties.

The Shiatsu Society is the licensing body for shiatsu. All practitioners on the register have passed the society's practical assessment. For a list of practitioners send an s.a.e. to the address on page 175.

Yoga

Yoga originated in India at least 3,000 years ago. It works in a holistic way – creating a general improvement in physical as well as mental well-being. There are three main elements: the practice of postures (*asanas*); breathing exercises (*pranayama*); and relaxation and concentration exercises. Yoga regains and maintains the suppleness of joints and relieves stress in those who are prone to stress–related headaches and migraines.

The British Wheel of Yoga is the largest yoga body in Britain and is also the co-ordinating body for local yoga groups. Lists of regional groups are obtainable from the society by writing to the address on page 175.

ADDRESSES

British Migraine Association
178a High Road, Byfleet, Weybridge, Surrey KT14 7ED
BYFLEET (0932) 352468

The Migraine Trust
45 Great Ormond Street, London WC1N 3HD
071-278 2676

Migraine clinics

The City of London Migraine Clinic
22 Charterhouse Square, London EC1M 6DX
071-251 3322
Will treat people without an appointment only during an acute attack. The clinic is a charity and treatment is free. Non-acute patients must have a referral letter from their GP.

King's College Hospital
Denmark Hill, London SE5 9RS
071-274 6222

Princess Margaret Migraine Clinic
Charing Cross Hospital, Fulham Palace Road, London W6 8RF
081-741 7833
Will treat people during acute attacks. A National Health Service clinic.

Many neurological departments in NHS hospitals will see migraine patients. The following hospitals will do so but patients must first obtain a referral letter from their GP.

LONDON
Elizabeth Garrett Anderson Hospital (*women only*)
144 Euston Road, London NW1 2AU
071-387 2501

Guy's Hospital
St Thomas Street, London SE1 9RT
071-407 7600

Hammersmith Hospital
150 Du Cane Road, Hammersmith, London W12 0HS
081-743 2030

The National Hospital for Neurology and Neurosurgery
Queen Square, London WC1N 3BG
071-837 3611

BELFAST
Claremont Street Hospital
Claremont Street, Belfast BT9 6AQ
BELFAST (0232) 40491

BIRMINGHAM
The Birmingham and Midland Eye Hospital
Church Street, Birmingham, West Midlands B3 2NS
BIRMINGHAM 021-236 4911

BRIGHTON
Royal Sussex County Hospital
Brighton, East Sussex BN2 5BE
BRIGHTON (0273) 606611

BRISTOL
Bristol Royal Infirmary
Bristol, Avon BS2 8HW
BRISTOL (0272) 22041

Bristol Royal Hospital for Sick Children
St Michael's Hill, Bristol, Avon BS2 8BJ
BRISTOL (0272) 215411

CAMBRIDGE
Addenbrooke's Hospital
Hills Road, Cambridge, Cambridgeshire CB2 2QQ
CAMBRIDGE (0223) 245151

EXETER
Royal Devon and Exeter Hospital
Barrack Road, Exeter, Devon EX2 5DW
EXETER (0392) 77833

GLASGOW
Institute of Neurological Sciences
Southern General Hospital, 1345 Govan Road, Glasgow G51 4TF
GLASGOW 041-445 2466

GUILDFORD
Farnham Road Hospital
Farnham Road, Guildford, Surrey GU2 5LX
GUILDFORD (0483) 571122

HARLOW
Princess Alexandra Hospital
Hamstel Road, Harlow, Essex CM20 1QX
HARLOW (0279) 26791

HARROW
Northwick Park Hospital
Watford Road, Harrow, Middlesex HA1 3UJ
081-864 5311

KINGSTON UPON HULL
Hull Royal Infirmary
Anlaby Road, Kingston upon Hull, North Humberside
HU3 2TZ
KINGSTON UPON HULL (0482) 28541

LEICESTER
Leicester Royal Infirmary
Leicester, Leicestershire LE1 5WW
LEICESTER (0533) 541414

LIVERPOOL
Regional Neurological Unit
Walton Hospital, Liverpool, Merseyside L9 1AE
LIVERPOOL 051-525 3611

Alder Hey Children's Hospital
Eaton Road, Liverpool, Merseyside L12 2AP
LIVERPOOL 051-228 4811

NEWCASTLE-UPON-TYNE
Regional Neurological Centre
Newcastle General Hospital, Westgate Road, Newcastle-upon-Tyne, Tyne and Wear NE4 6BE
NEWCASTLE-UPON-TYNE 091–273 8811

NOTTINGHAM
General Hospital
Park Row, Nottingham, Nottinghamshire NG7 2UH
NOTTINGHAM (0602) 481100

NUNEATON
George Eliot Hospital
College Street, Nuneaton, Warwickshire CV10 7DG
NUNEATON (0203) 384201

OXFORD
John Radcliffe Hospital II (*for children only*)
Paediatric Unit, Headington, Oxford, Oxfordshire OX2 6HE
OXFORD (0865) 64711

PRESTON
Preston Royal Infirmary
Preston, Lancashire PR1 6PS
PRESTON (0772) 716565

ROMFORD
Regional Centre for Neurology
Oldchurch Hospital, Oldchurch Road, Romford, Essex RM7 0BE
ROMFORD (0708) 460909

SOUTHAMPTON
Southampton General Hospital
Shirley, Southampton, Hampshire SO9 4XY
SOUTHAMPTON (0703) 777222

SOUTHEND
Southend Hospital
Prittlewell Chase, Westcliff-on-Sea, Essex SS0 0RY
SOUTHEND (0702) 348911

Complementary therapies

The following list of representative bodies is not exhaustive. Space permits only a small number of these in existence to be mentioned here.

ACUPUNCTURE
British Medical Acupuncture Society
Newton House, Newton Lane, Lower Whitley, Warrington, Cheshire WA4 4JA
WARRINGTON (092) 573727

The College of Traditional Chinese Acupuncture
Tao House, Queensway, Leamington Spa, Warwickshire CV31 3LZ
LEAMINGTON SPA (0926) 22121
(for the training of lay acupuncturists)

ALEXANDER TECHNIQUE
The Society of Teachers of the Alexander Technique (STAT)
10 London House, 266 Fulham Road, London SW10 9EL
071-351 0828

AROMATHERAPY
International Federation of Aromatherapists
4 Eastmearn Road, West Dulwich, London SE21 8HA

CHIROPRACTIC
British Chiropractic Association
Premier House, 10 Greycoat Place, London SW1P 1SB
071-222 8866

HOMOEOPATHY
British Homoeopathic Association
27a Devonshire Street, London W1N 1RJ
071-935 2163

Society of Homoeopaths
2 Artizan Road, Northampton, Northamptonshire NN1 4HU
NORTHAMPTON (0604) 21400

HOMOEOPATHIC HOSPITALS WITHIN THE NATIONAL HEALTH SERVICE

The Royal London Homoeopathic Hospital
Great Ormond Street, London WC1N 3HR
071-837 3091

Glasgow Homoeopathic Hospital
1000 Great Western Road, Glasgow G12 0YN
GLASGOW 041-339 0382

Outpatient Clinic for Adults and Children
The Old Health Institute, Buchanan Street, Baillieston, Glasgow G69 6DA
GLASGOW 041-771 7396

Mossley Hill Hospital
Park Avenue, Liverpool, Merseyside L18 8BU
LIVERPOOL 051-724 2335

Bristol Homoeopathic Hospital
Cotham, Bristol, Avon BS6 6JU
BRISTOL (0272) 731231

CLINIC NOT IN THE NATIONAL HEALTH SERVICE

The Manchester Homoeopathic Clinic
Brunswick Street, Ardwick, Manchester M13 9ST
MANCHESTER 061-273 2446

MEDICAL HERBALISM
National Institute of Medical Herbalists
9 Palace Gate, Exeter, Devon EX1 1JA
EXETER (0392) 426022

OSTEOPATHY
The General Council and Register of Osteopaths
56 London Street, Reading, Berks RG1 4SQ
READING (0734) 576585

REFLEXOLOGY
The British School of Reflexology
92 Sheering Road, Old Harlow, Essex CM17 0JW
HARLOW (0279) 429060

SHIATSU
Shiatsu Society, 14 Oakdene Road, Redhill, Surrey RH1 6BT
REDHILL (0737) 767896 (1-4pm)

YOGA
The British Wheel of Yoga
1 Hamilton Place, Boston Road, Sleaford, Lincolnshire
NG34 7ES
SLEAFORD (0529) 306851

The Biomedical Trust
PO Box 140, Cambridge, Cambridgeshire CB1 1PU

FURTHER READING

Blau, J. N., ed. *Migraine: clinical, therapeutic, conceptual and research aspects*, London, Chapman and Hall, 1987

Kudrow, L., *Cluster Headaches Mechanism & Management*, New York and London, OUP, 1980

Lance, J. W., *Mechanism and Management of Headache (fourth ed.)*, London, Butterworth, 1982

Sachs, O., *Migraine: Understanding the Common Disorder*, London, Pan, 1985

INDEX